Praise for A Healing Mind

Dr. Kuhn's memoir moved me deeply. It inspired me so much; I had to read it two times. Even though many Chinese experienced the cultural revolution, not many had her unique experience, courage, endurance, determination, and positive attitude. I highly recommend people of any age, especially younger folks, read this book to be inspired and to be successful in their career.

----Mandy Wang, China

Aihan's memoir is plain, ordinary, and extraordinary. The whole book displays her courage, bravery, facing the challenges of life's journey. It is an inspirational journey and an inspirational girl who set a learning model for all of us and all generations. The realistic atmosphere is the highlight of the memoir. For Aihan, thumbs up!

---- Bingqing Zhao, Professor, Hunan University of Traditional Chinese Medicine

Dr. Kuhn's story is one of struggle, growth, and achievement. While providing an eye-opening look back at a difficult time for many people in the fledgling Chinese Republic, it also illustrates the thirst for opportunity and dogged determination that seems so prevalent in the Chinese character. Dr. Kuhn has genuinely "lived and learned" and happily shares her experience, hoping that we might all benefit from the telling.

----Gerry Kuhn

Praise for A Healing Mind continued...

I first met Aihan on March 1, 1978. As a "day student," I came to the school dining hall to have breakfast. At that time, the students all dressed in plain clothes, we all looked young, and between the opposite sex, they dare not face each other directly. Our group had 11 people, male six, female five, (originally it was five male five female, but I was a "day student" added to our group, I felt the loss of "Yin and Yang balance." I sat between them busying myself with eating, occasionally looking at my classmates in the group, female classmates wore braided hairstyles almost everyone, showing their youth.

One temperamental female was different from the other girls. When she was talking and smiling, there were small dimples on the corners of her mouth; later, I learned that she was Aihan. At that time, we (especially girls), all young and bashful, dare not speak, especially dare not look at the boys. We were all absorbed in reading; rarely would female students have opportunities to communicate. Over time, we had a little better understanding of each other; we were a little bit more casual, too. When I first started school, I dressed in some of the most tattered clothes you might ever see. I wore corduroy tops and patched khaki pants. Many students came from rural areas and had made new clothes to study in the city. However, most of them dressed in blue, gray, or black. Most of them wore students' clothes and "Mao" suits.

Before long, the secretary saw that I was "poor" and sent me an application form for "financial aid." After filling in the application form, I did not get any financial aid. Later, I learned that many students from rural areas were in tough circumstances and needed to get financial assistance. Aihan and Zhang Yi and I did not get financial aid. Later, I found out that Aihan's family condition was relatively good at that time, belonging to the "red second generation." Her temperament was different from that of our other female classmates. She was always smiling, unashamed, natural, singing and dancing, and was a well-educated, literate, intellectual lady who always "rolled her eyes" when speaking to others, making the boys roll their eyes. Literature and art class activities, she was always there, like a literary youth. However, she had a simple personality and was outspoken, which inevitably led to some "domineering" sounding speech. Therefore, several interested members of the opposite sex, had their interest "nipped in the bud."

 I remember the first summer vacation (summer of 1978), our grade participated in the school's "air defense system" project. Our group was assigned in front of the old library in a space to dig down, about 4 meters deep, we began to dig, here the sand and gravel was soft but not easy to dig. After digging about 60 to 70CM horizontally, everyone took a rest. Aihan and several classmates climbed the stairs to the ground level to rest. I thought it should be more relaxed in the hole, so I stayed alone in the trench. A while later, Aihan called me up to rest, I was not willing to go, thinking it more refreshing below, but Aihan told me there was wind above, initially feeling cool I suddenly felt hot, suddenly sweating, after a minute I also followed them to ground level. Less than five minutes later, my original resting place appeared to collapse; this gave me a cold sweat, Aihan had saved me!

---- Changgang Li, Director of Internal Medicine of Pediatrics Department, Shenzhen Children's Hospital

A Healing Mind Moving through Life

The Amazing Journey of a Holistic Doctor

Dr. Aihan Kuhn

Copyright © 2020 Dr. Aihan Kuhn

All rights reserved.

ISBN-13: 979-8-63066-904-9

Contents

Foreword i
Preface iii
Acknowledgment: v
Introduction vi
PART I: A LONG JOURNEY IN CHINA 1
Chapter 1: Childhood Memories 3
Chapter 2: Cultural Revolution 11
Chapter 3: Moving from City to Town 21
Chapter 4: Memorable Farm Life 27
Chapter 5: Easier Farm Life 43
Chapter 6: Busy Life in Medical School 49
Chapter 7: Practicing Medicine 55
Chapter 8: The Pursuit of Love 59
Chapter 9: Unfortunate Life 63
Chapter 10: Keep Learning and Life Changes 71
PART II: A CHALLENGING JOURNEY IN THE USA 79
Chapter 11: Living in the States 81
Chapter 12: Journey to Holistic Medicine 95
Chapter 13: Non-Profit Work 109
PART III: WHAT I LEARNED AND WHAT I GAINED 129
Chapter 14: Learning from Mistakes & Slip-ups 131
Chapter 15: Learn to be a Good Leader 137
Chapter 16: Embrace and Cherish Cultural Differences 141
Chapter 17: About My Father 167
Chapter 18: My Hip Story 177
PART IV   TIPS FOR HAPPINESS AND SUCCESS 185
Chapter 19: What Brings True Happiness? 187
Chapter 20: Valuable Tips for Success in Life and Career ... 203
Chapter 21: Good Health, East Meets West 225

I dedicate this book to my husband, Gerry Kuhn, my daughter Sharon Kuhn, and my son Peter Kuhn. My love for you is deep and forever.

--- Aihan Kuhn

Foreword

Here is the memoir of Dr. Aihan Kuhn. She lived through a chaotic period in Chinese history and then faced a challenging new culture living in the United States. She was born in China and lived there for 30 years, now living in the United States (for 30 years). She experienced much turmoil and confusion and a destructive period during the cultural revolution. She witnessed family chaos and experienced a difficult life in the countryside, along with many other teenagers. She had both personal loss and gain, but these experiences helped to build her character. Her desire to go to school fulfilled when she is finally able to study medicine in medical school.

Trained in conventional medicine in China Dr. Kuhn then came to the United States in 1989, she experienced many differences in life, society, work, culture, daily activities, customs, food, mindset, etiquette, and more. She endured many challenges and obstacles, experienced many changes and much healing, and grew into an extraordinary person. Dr. Kuhn always learned and studied to build her career and learned to adapt to a different culture and become a well-known holistic doctor, healer, master teacher of Qi Gong and Tai Chi, and an award-winning author. She has helped many others to heal, to grow, and to succeed.

Her personal life and health had also gone through turmoil, but with wisdom, practice, and constant learning, she has been able to restore harmony, happiness, and balanced life.

Sharing her experience with what works and what doesn't work, she provides "Golden Tips for Success and Life-Long Happiness." These may significantly benefit not only adults but also the younger generation who want to succeed in life and career.

She set a paradigm/model for holistic practitioners, therapists, and medical doctors. She was the owner of Chinese Medicine for Health, New England School of Tai Chi (closed after she moved to Florida). She is the President of Tai Chi & Qi Gong Healing Institute, a non-profit organization promoting natural health, healing, a stress-free lifestyle, and lifelong happiness. She has gone on from being a non-English speaker to becoming a speaker, award-winning author, and master teacher. She has come a long way.

From her innocent upbringing during the turbulent years of the Cultural Revolution, to her back-breaking work as a field hand, to her establishment of a new life and successful holistic healing business in America, she then becomes an award-winning author. Aihan's indomitable spirit shines through it all.

Preface

Why am I writing about this life journey? Every one of us has beautiful life stories, but not everyone is willing to put in the time to record these stories. As we get older, our memory declines, our brain's storage space becomes smaller. Our mind is limited, but our life experience is not limited. Many beautiful memories (and some not so beautiful ones that can be life lessons), and valuable life experiences can be lost if we don't write them down. By reading our stories, the next generation may avoid our mistakes, and they may have a better and smoother journey than us.

By writing down events and lessons in our lives, we can continue to grow no matter how young or how old we are. At least to me, because I pay more attention to English language structure through writing, it helps my English skills.

I started to write this book in 1994. Not only did I have the experience of living in two different countries, two different cultures, and two separate educational systems, I also worked in various medical fields. At that time, my spiritual growth followed an ancient philosophy. I decided to organize all of this by putting it into a book. Hopefully, it will benefit some people or the next generation. I started to put my stories together, and I thought if I don't do this now, my story may be lost. I cannot remember everything, but some critical pieces that either traumatized me or rewarded me can be educational or inspirational.

In 2002 or 2003, (I forget the exact year), after I had completed about a third of writing my story, I asked a publisher if it would be worth it to write a biography and if they would be interested in publishing this kind of book. The answer I got was: "It will not sell unless you are dead." That was discouraging!

So, I paused in completing this book. But since I had already written nearly half, I decided to put some of the chapters into my newsletter with each newsletter containing one story. My "fans" (my students and my patients) loved my stories and told me they could not wait for the next newsletter. That was encouraging! So, I got my balance!

After many years of teaching, helping patients get well, and writing numerous other books, I built up more credibility and had more "true fans." Some former students who had seen the chapters in my newsletters began asking me when I would be finishing the book. I finally decided to complete this project, or otherwise, all my work would be lost. Time is precious, and I hated the idea of wasting all the time I had spent on this project before. I know it is a lot of work to complete a book, but hopefully, my readers will enjoy it, or some readers may learn from my mistakes. I am not great at the English language, but at least I can tell stories about my life and my healing experiences.

As English is my second language, I know I can never be perfect at it, especially since we lose our abilities as we are getting older. But, as long as I continue to read, to write, and to speak, I can always improve. Writing is one of the many ways to keep our brain active. I am still learning new words and how to use them correctly. One of my books published in 2008, Simple Chinese Medicine, got an award, third place in the US best book category in Holistic healing. I cannot believe I became an "Award-Winning Author." In 2017, three of my books were nominated "Best books" in different categories. These books are Brain Fitness, Tai Chi in 10 Weeks, and Tai Chi for Depression.

In April 2019, I found out that my book True Wellness co-written with Dr. Kurosu, had received two awards in three different categories: medicine, health, and nutrition. The awards are in both content and title. The truth is: the less I expect, the more I get.

I realize the more I write, the better I get. All my students and my patients enjoy my books, and they are inspired by reading them to do better in self-care and try to improve their quality of life.

----Aihan Kuhn, 2019

Acknowledgment:

To write this memoir took many days and nights trying to recall information about my life stories from deep within my memory storage. I had nearly forgotten many of my early life stories; But thanks to many of the people who were on the path with me, I was able to retrieve a lot of them.

My gratitude goes out to my friends in the countryside, my classmates (class 8) from medical school, and my family members: my sisters and brothers, who provided valuable memories in parts of experiences I couldn't remember. I also want to thank my husband, Gerry, who did the first edit to check the grammar and language. Special thanks to my older sister, who helped me correct the Chinese language version using translation software from the internet. I also want to thank my fans and my students, who encouraged me to complete this memoir.

Introduction

Having lived in the US for 30 years, I have to say I am a lucky woman, for many reasons. I feel fortunate to have a wonderful family: my husband, my two beautiful children, and my wonderful family in China. I feel lucky that I have achieved all I had dreamed of; I feel fortunate to have so many fans all over the country and in other countries too. I feel lucky that so many people enjoy reading my books even though I am still trying to learn English in both speaking and writing, and I know I can never be perfect. I feel lucky to have so many supporters. I'm grateful to my students, patients, friends, my fans all over the world, and my family in China.

As an immigrant, I did not take any jobs from Americans. Instead, I have created jobs for others. I never took any government help even in my most challenging time when I was beginning my life in the US. And I have paid taxes all the while, and I have worked hard just like many others.

I am grateful for everything, including the kind help of so many lovely people. But my strength came from my life journey. I never try intentionally to brag about myself in my writing, but here I will share some unforgettable stories that I experienced. I have no expectations about how people may react, but considering the excellent feedback I had from people who read my other books, I guess I am doing something right. Therefore, I am presenting the limited memories from my brain, putting them into words so that maybe my readers will be entertained and can enjoy passing some time reading.

Every morning I wake up and walk out into the backyard, listening to the birds talking to each other, squirrels chasing each other, I look at my garden and smell my Jasmine and Gardenia flowers, a sense of joy goes through my whole body. I don't want to leave my garden, but I remember I have to finish my books, especially this memoir.

2019 is a fantastic year for me for several reasons. It is my 30th anniversary of living in the United States. One of my books (from the medical book series), which I co-wrote with Dr. Kurosu, got two book awards. Living in Florida and loving orchids, many of my orchids are blooming this year. (but I lost so in the past many because I am still learning how to grow them) My non-profit, "Tai Chi & Qi Gong Healing Institute," got more new members than any other year. And my husband retired this year. This year is the People's Republic of China's 70th birthday (1949 to 2019), and I have seen so many changes in the Chinese lifestyle, technology, and economic development.

It seems like a special year. So, I'm inspired to complete this book; as a gift to my family, friends, fans, and my readers.

Born and raised in China, I experienced various turbulent times and went through all kinds of emotional and physical struggles. I finally found my way, which is to tap into the calm solitude, peace, and harmony that already exists inside me. However, it is not easy to open myself up and share these personal stories in writing with the public, especially some of the super old memories. But after seeing so many patients who suffer from emotional and physical issues, and many of them so unhappy with their life, observing some of the confusion that my kids face, I felt this memoir might cheer them up. Maybe they may feel grateful for not having to go through as much as I did, or perhaps it might provide some insight or guidance if they read this memoir. For the younger generation, I hope to inspire them, especially my children.

Part I: A Long Journey in China

Chapter 1: Childhood Memories

When I was a little girl, I always dreamed that I could fly in the sky, with no fear, no worry, and free of everything. When I was about 5 or 6 years old, I asked myself, "why can birds fly, but we cannot?" "What if I jump from a big rock and wave my arms, can I fly then?" "Would a rabbit understand me if I talked to them?" I had so many questions about nature, about plants, about creatures. Whenever I had the chance, I often walked in the fields where there were a lot of wildflowers, weeds, grass, and stones. I often looked at the sky, listened to the birds singing, breathing in the fresh air, and catching some grasshoppers, dragonflies, and butterflies.

I usually picked some fresh wildflowers and smelled them, then put some in my hair. I then looked into the water to see the reflection: it is like a mirror! I look pretty! I sometimes thought I was in a movie, and someone is filming me to record everything I was doing. Those were my special innocent times. I love nature! I love being with nature; I love everything that view offers to me. I can feel the power of life, and I always feel good when I am outside with nature for many reasons. I can feel the love from nature. I feel nature hugging me, holding me, making me so cozy, warm, and comfortable. I felt so good when I was out there even if it was raining. Somedays, I did not mind being by myself, although I love to play with other kids. It was always hard to say good-bye when I left the field to go back home.

When I was about 11 years old, I cut a willow tree branch then put in the ground behind my parent's apartment because I want to see if this branch could grow to a tree. I watered it every day and observed it grew every day. Surprisingly to me, this branch became a small willow tree one year later. Ever since then, I became interested in growing things, not that I had any knowledge about how to grow anything. But I would put some soil in a broken dish, then pick some wildflowers put them in the soil, and watch it to see if the flowers could survive. Of course, as it was, most of them failed. The older I got, the more I am drawn to nature, even to the point I became a doctor of natural medicine.

I grew up in a large, very strict family. My father and mother were in the Army during World War II fighting the Japanese. During that time, my father participated in the war, but my mother was assigned doing the work of logistic support. Also, this was about the time my two sisters were born (1947, 1949). After the communist takeover of China in 1949, my mother retired from the Army and was assigned to study in college; she studied finance and economics. She later worked in banks (several different banks over time). In 1950, my father went to the Korean War as a battalion commander (But I did not get a chance asking my father about those stories may be in part because I was not interested at that time). The war lasted for a year, and he returned home in 1951.

After the Korean War, my father was sent to a military cadre school to study politics in Chang Chun, and later, he was teaching in the same school. In 1960, my father went to the Military University of Political Science in Beijing, and he studied political science from 1960 to 1963. After graduating in 1963, our whole family moved to Changsha because my father was assigned to teach in a military cadre school of political science in Changsha.

My family lived at the military college. We lived in an apartment complex provided to teachers. At that time, my father was a teacher in this military college specializing in education that produced political leaders in the military. This military college community was gated, with a military guard 24/7. There were buildings of classrooms, practice grounds for soldiers to practice shooting, a dormitory for military students, and apartment housing for teachers and their families. There were some grassy areas not developed, and this was how I took advantage of going there with other kids about my age or a little older. Sometimes I would even go there by myself.

My parents were terrific people, kind, giving, and always willing to help others when needed. In my family, there are six of us, and I am number five. The first three are girls three years apart, then my older brother two years older than me, and my younger brother two years younger. All my siblings have particular strengths: my oldest sister is intelligent and has a logical mind; my second sister is hard-working and kind, always helping others; my third sister is frugal and doesn't waste anything, and cares about other people; my older brother has a fantastic personality, patient, and has excellent social skills; my younger brother is multi-talented, good with people and also has excellent social skills. I am number five, a little quiet, shy, but stubborn in some ways.

We were told by our parents to study hard in school and work hard at home; be a good person and always be honest in any situation; help other people not just think of our self; love our country and do anything for our country. Both of my parents were working and busy. Therefore, my father had a unique way of making my sisters do the housework: five cents (Chinese cents) for dishes, ten cents for cleaning the floor, and ten cents babysitting my younger brother and me. Each of them had a job, and it worked! The housework got done, and no one complained. We did not realize this was a type of "capitalist" motivation.

I was stubborn and brave. I remember one day, my grandmother and my mother blamed me for the loss of 5 yuan (Chinese dollars). At that time, five Chinese dollars was a good chunk of money. I was furious because I did not take the money, nor did I know anything about where their money was. They insisted that I must have taken this money, no matter how much I explained that I was innocent. My mother spanked me, that was like putting oil over the fire. I knew there was no way to make them believe me, and I was distraught, so I ran out of my home. It was pouring outside, and I had no umbrella. I ran and ran, crying all the way. I thought the world was unfair and so difficult, especially when no one would believe that I was an honest girl. I was hurt badly.

At that moment, I wished that I came from a different family, a family that believed me, loved me and supported me. I decided not to go back home. But where could I go? The answer was nowhere.

Finally, one of my sisters found me outside of our apartment building, under the roof. She asked me to go back home and apologize to my mother. Her point was that no matter what, I should not run away from home. I said "no" in the beginning, then I gave up and followed my sister home. Later, I realized I was stupid and stubborn. But as I have been thinking back, there was no way I could prove my innocence.

At the beginning of 1966, my father retired from the military teaching job and was assigned to work in the Bureau of Agriculture Development. Since my father was in a higher position, he got an apartment with four rooms, while most families only had two rooms. Within the four rooms, one was the kitchen, one was the dining room, and also where my two brothers slept, one bedroom for my parents, and one bedroom for four girls. Fortunately, two of my sisters lived at school most of the time.

We used a coal stove to cook meals. Cooking is a long process; you can imagine using one stove for cooking for a family of six to eight people. Waiting for dinner to be ready was always tough. We washed the vegetables using a water source outside in the back of the house that we shared with four other families. I remember in wintertime, when the temperature dropped below 30 degrees, the pipes would freeze, and we could not get the water out. We sometimes had to put water in a big ceramic container that could hold 10 gallons of water in case the pipe froze, and we were not able to get water. I often washed vegetables in a basin outside with no gloves. During winter, the cold water made my hands turn from red to purple, and my body felt like I was in an ice cave. It felt like a thousand knives stabbing into my bones. This extremely unpleasant feeling made me cry sometimes. I was only ten or eleven years old. I prayed whenever I was using cold water: please give me some warm water. I would sometimes boil water then mix it in with the cold water to escape the extreme cold. My hands often chapped, even bleeding sometimes no matter how many times I put Vaseline type ointment on them. It was nobody's fault, it was just a reality of life, and there was nothing anyone could do.

I was an outgoing child and always had a lot of friends in my neighborhood. I was brave, laughed loud, had my own ideas of how to play: sometimes dolls, make-believe cooking, jumping rope, sometimes cards, and sometimes we would draw on the paved road then jump over from one square to another. We fought occasionally, but shortly afterward, we were back playing. I always fought and defended the weak against bullies and helped the kid who was in need. I always tried to do the right thing.

Our elementary school was impoverished with broken chairs and tables. The roof would sometimes leak when it was raining, and the floor was muddy. The school management was poor. The teachers didn't care much about how the kids behaved outside the classroom; they were there to teach. There was no such thing as a school counselor. Outside the school, the children fought a lot. I remember one day I fought with my friend. She had a bad mouth and always told lies and caused trouble. I yelled at her, and I may have pushed her. I don't remember exactly. The next day she brought her brother to my class, and her brother beat me up. I was upset and went home and told the whole story to my brother, who was two years older than me. My brother was older and bigger than my friend's brother. Three days later, my brother came to my school and beat up her brother outside of school and told him not to touch me again. On the fourth day, her brother beat me up again! I realized it was a mistake to continue this cycle. I didn't tell my brother this time. I started wondering why this happened. After that, I never told my brother what happened in school. I realized if I had stopped in the first place, things would have been much better, and nobody would have gotten hurt. I guess I learned the hard way.

We were often short of food such as rice, flour, and other things. Each family received a fixed amount of tickets (liang piao) from the government for rice and flour, depending on how many people were in the family. We still had to pay for some things. But we had plenty of sweet potatoes (hong shu), there was no shortage of them. My parents bought so many sweet potatoes; we had to eat them every day in various ways of cooking: steamed, fried, boiled, baked, dried, mixed in rice, in porridge, in soup…. Oh my God, any way to cook a sweet potato that my family could think up. I was so tired of eating sweet potatoes that I never wanted to eat them again after that.

    We didn't always have good food, but every Chinese New Year, we put on a big feast. I would often eat so much that I got sick. My mind was made up to eat as much as I could because I knew there would be other times when I would not have these tasty foods. Every Chinese New Year, I got sick to my stomach and threw up. I think I may still have this habit of overeating around the holidays. Most of the time, we ate our whole meal with nothing leftover. Occasionally though, there was sometimes a bit of leftover food on the dining table covered with screened net. At that time, there was no refrigerator, and leftover food would remain on the table. I often got up in the middle of the night stealing some food to feed myself, luckily no one knew. Those years no one focuses on nutrition, or good flavor food, nor variety; we only concentrated on not being hungry. My parents rarely bought snacks for us, but sometimes they would get popcorn from a vendor who carries "Pop machine" on the street, made popcorn right there. This how it works: we brought one pound of rice or corn to the vender when we heard the bell sound (from vendor), pay 10 cents (Chinese cents), the vender would pop for us. We then ended up with a massive bag of snacks.

    Later, when I was a teenager, my parents gave me some money, I would spend it for a bowl of rice noodles, which was so delicious and cheap. I still like this dish, and every time I go back to China, I always go into a restaurant to eat a bowl of rice noodles. I highly recommend anyone who gets a chance to go to Changsha; try a bowl of rice noodles, but don't be afraid of adding some hot pepper.

☐

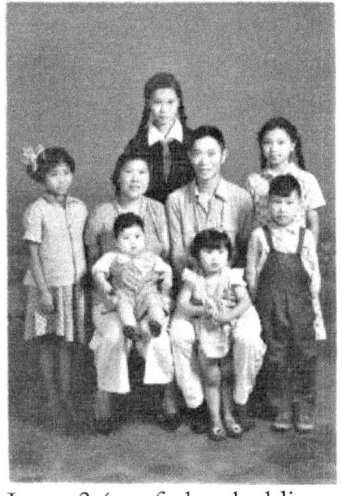 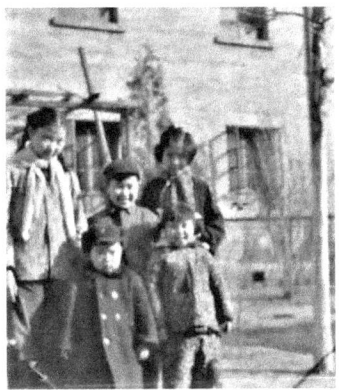

1. I was 3 (my father holding me).
2. I was 5, the first row on the right, in Changchun, NE China

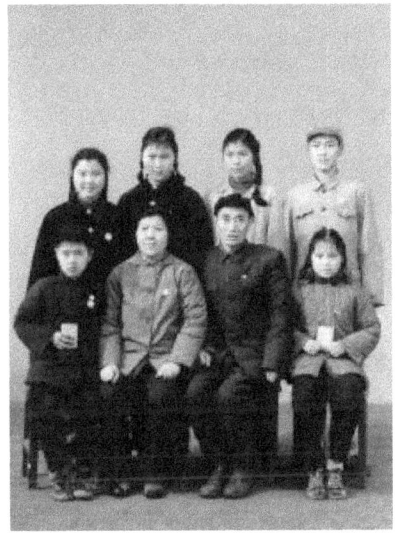 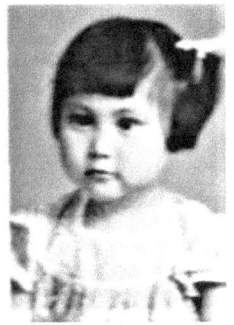

3. 1968 holding a "Redbook"
4. I was three years old

Chapter 2: Cultural Revolution

About May 1966, the famous "Chinese Cultural Revolution" started. The nightmare began. The Cultural Revolution, as it was officially known, was a 10-year social, political movement initiated to strengthen Maoism in China by eliminating capitalist, feudalistic, and cultural elements through an ideological campaign aimed at reviving revolutionary spirit and purging the country of "impure" elements. An internal power struggle quickly spilled over into all facets of society. Destruction and violence of unspeakable proportions ensued. This shocking movement intended to create a new culture by destroying traditional beliefs, customs, and thinking, by purging "revisionist thought" and by crushing perceived enemies of the Communist Party. These ten years (when I was 10 to 20 years old) are the most critical decades in my personal growth, learning, searching, trying to figure things out, and choose my path. But I was totally at a loss with such a turbulent time, a confused mind, and damaged spirit.

In 1966 Mao had called on the student Red Guards to rebel against "reactionary" authorities. He aimed to reshape society by purging it of bourgeois elements and traditional ways of thinking. Millions of people were arrested and terrorized by the Red Guards, the Cultural Revolution's paramilitary youth organization. Those detained were forced to endure brutal "struggle sessions," where they were tortured and humiliated in public. By the summer of 1968, the country was engulfed in fighting, as Red Guard factions competed for power. By the time the revolution ended in 1976, as many as three million people had been killed.

At that time, students had to stop going to school, get out of the classroom to fight, to protect the communist party, protect "Chairman Mao," to become a "Red Guard." The posters and banners were all over the place. The loud-speakers were so loud, and you could hear it every minute, sometimes even when you were sleeping. The Red Guard was everywhere; they wore military clothes and a red arm-band, so people would recognize that they were "good people" and "fighters for Chairman Mao" and the communist government. There were many different kinds of Red Guards. Some were gentle, and some were violent and brutal. Three of my sisters joined the Red Guard; they were in a "Gentle Red Guard" group. They thought they were protecting Chairman Mao; they felt they were doing good things. I was too little to join, but I joined "the little Red Guard" (I was ten years old). We were asked to send out flyers, to read the "Red book" on the street, and to parade in the road holding the national flag. Everyone was acting crazy, had no clue what we were doing, or what was going on, but did what we were told to do. I saw many Red Guard dance on the street; they had a special dance, nothing like any dance we knew. I often heard gunshots, feeling chaotic, disorganized, did not know what was going on. Sometimes we heard there were bodies on the street.

The Red Guard traveled many places on the train free of charge or with a discounted ticket. They sometimes got free food and a free room when they visited another city with a similar group of Red guards. Some groups of "Red Guard" would go to people's houses and break things saying that they were "Old stuff," "Yellow stuff," "anti-Revolution stuff." Some of them stole people's jewelry saying "jewelry is garbage," a "capitalist product." They took "well-known people" out of their homes, and put them on the street or stage, hung a big wood board on their neck, made them kneel on the ground. They told people that these "well-known people," "Educated people" were "anti-Revolution" and "Capitalism-Followers." Red guards sometimes brutally beat them and kicked them.

One day, coming home from a friend's house, I saw the crowds on the basketball court. I walked close by and saw my father and several other people who were also in higher positions were kneeling on the floor of the stage about 3 or 4 feet above the ground, with big board hanging on their necks. My father had a good job with higher pay than average. He was a small leader in the "New Fourth Army" (Xin Si Jun) during World War II while fighting the Japanese in China. Then he went to Army College after the liberation of China in 1949. He started teaching at Army College in the early '60s. He had position, education, and life experience. But no matter what kind person he was, he could not escape being accused because 90% of people with higher rank, top leaders, educated people were accused of whatever nonsense reason that the Red Guard could give. This stupid movement swept up even senior government officials.

My heart was broken, and I ran home as fast as I could. I didn't want to see the details; I didn't want to see what was next. That evening my father came home did not say anything; the whole family did not talk. Dinner was silent; no one said anything. I was full of anger and had millions of questions about why and what was going on. Those days my parents were fighting very often, but I didn't know why. Later my sister told me that the Red guard and other groups forced my mother say bad things about my father so that they would have evidence against my father. My mother was forced to say something about my father. (I don't think it was my mother's fault, nobody can think clearly at that time, everyone was crazy.)

My father had been accused. Now the kids around my neighborhood were quite mean to my younger brothers and me. My older brother and sisters were out all the time, left at home was my younger brother and me. They threw stones to our windows, called us names using bad language, threw rocks or stones at my younger brother and me; they said we came from a bad family, we were terrible people. I fought a lot with them, but I could not win because I was just one, and they were so many. Often, I came home with a bruise on my face, arms, or legs, and dirty clothes. The anger in me was getting worse; I was not happy and did not know what happiness meant. Maybe there was no such thing as "Happiness." My younger brother and I used to fight a lot, but when other kids bully us, he and I put energy together to fight against these kids.

Later in life, when I studied medicine, especially learning Chinese Medicine, I realized my liver had some significant imbalance, most likely situational: too many negative experiences, too much anger.

During the Cultural Revolution, many companies closed. All schools closed; students were out on the street, teachers either hiding, or stayed in the house not going out, and did not dare to say anything. There were many gunfights and fistfights. It was chaos. Since all the schools in Changsha City were closed, my parents decided to send my brother, who was two years younger, and me, to Shanghai, where we were still able to go to school. Shanghai school system was not affected by the Cultural Revolution, even though there was some chaos too. While we were in Shanghai, we stayed with my aunt and my grandparents.

Shanghai is the biggest city in China, like New York City in the United States. There was also a lot of fighting in Shanghai but less than in Changsha, where my parents lived. My brother and I attended school in Shanghai for one year. I was in third grade, my brother in first. The school was fine. At that time, Shanghai people disliked people from different cities or different provinces; they believe they were better than others. The kids in school were not friendly at all. That did not bother me because I knew I would eventually go back home to Changsha.

I lived with my aunt and uncle with their three children (ages 2, 4, 8) and my grandfather, grandmother — all in a two-bedroom apartment, with seven people living there. But now, after my younger brother and I moved in, nine people were living in this two-bedroom apartment. My aunt's whole family were living in one bedroom; my Grandparents and I, with my younger brother, lived in the other bedroom. The kitchen was so small that we only had a small table for meals, not much space to walk around. It was a bit crowded.

My grandfather was very strict and stubborn. I called him a tyrant. He made me, my brother, and my cousin read the "Red Book" every day. The "Red Book" was written by Chairman Mao, who had been ruling China from 1949 until the end of cultural revolution. We read the "Red Book" every day, and we were required to memorized a page per day. The "Red Book" seems like "Chinese Bible" that everyone must study and learn, as well as use in daily life. Some sayings in the book were logical, and some were not. I didn't care much for it because it was just too dull.

One day I got a stick beating from my grandfather because I did not read the Red book. I was angry. I took a big page from a newspaper and wrote with a Chinese paintbrush in black ink: "Grandfather is a tyrant, mean person, I will not obey you." I was an 11-year-old girl. I posted my sign on the front door so every neighbor passing by could see it. I was prepared to get a more significant spanking. Surprisingly, I didn't. My grandfather laughed after he saw this. My whole family was surprised that I did this. I was fearless but stupid; I was upset but also a little scared. My grandfather did not beat me this time but told me I still had to read the "Red Book" because it was the family rule. Wow, that was a little scary! But I needed to speak up for myself. From that age, I was searching for freedom.

In later years, my family and neighbors always used this as a joke; they teased me many times. My family and neighbors always said, "Aihan is so smart, she will be successful whatever she does." They did admire me for being "Fearless," "going for my goal."

I did not have much emotional attachment with my grandfather, but I loved my grandmother dearly, and I miss her forever. She was different, the kindest person I had ever known. She was a Buddhist, did not eat any meat, but later ate eggs, milk, and fish because she had a health issue and bone loss. She was very gentle, always ask grandfather not to be so hard on the children. She taught me a lot. She had tiny little feet and walked very slow. In old China, a family would bind a girl's feet starting at the age of three. The ancient China thought women with little feet looked more elegant, pretty; on the other hand, they did not want women to run away if the marriage did not work out. I sometimes saw my grandmother massage her feet; I knew her feet hurt. She was such a good cook and cooked for the whole family, but she did not eat much. I loved her pork dumplings, and I would always ask her to give me one before dinner. Every day she got up early to go to the market and get vegetables and meat for the family meals. She never complained, no matter what. She was very patient, tolerant, forgiving, and kind-hearted.

    Living in Shanghai for one year, I learned from my grandmother and my aunt how to sew, how to knit, how to do embroidery, and learned to speak Shanghai language (the language in China can be very different in different cities or provinces). I learned how to wash dishes, clean vegetables, some basic cooking, how to use a sewing machine. I even learned to make my clothes: made one shirt but stitched the collar wrong (stitched collar inside out), and sewed the right sleeve on left side of the shirt and stitched the left sleeve on right side of the shirt. I enjoyed being with my aunt, uncle, my grandmother, and my three cousins. In Shanghai, the lifestyle is a little different from Changsha. The neighbors are very friendly, very close, and visit each other very often. They often give each other homemade food. I got to taste different dishes. Neighbors gossip all the time when they visit each other; they enjoyed this social exchange, and it seemed very harmonious to me. Rarely did I see neighbors fighting; I only knew one neighbor who did not talk much to others. But if I initiated the conversation, they were fine and had no problem talking to me. After one year of living in Shanghai, I went back home to Changsha. I miss Shanghai a lot, and mostly I miss my Shanghai family, especially my grandmother and my aunt. I also miss my cousins; they always would accompany me anywhere I went, and we played together every day.

    I've always loved art, any art. I had a pleasant voice and enjoyed singing. Since I was chubby (in other words: fat), physically, I was not as agile as other kids. I did not do well in Physical Education class because I was too heavy. I hated my body, which was one of the big deals that affected my self-esteem. When I was 13 years old, my friends and I heard that there was an audition from a Hunan Folk Art performing company (Hua Gu Xi Ju Tuan), run by the province. They were looking for young actresses and singers. My friends and I decided to go for an audition. We went there and saw about 20 kids waiting outside the audition room. The audition required dancing and singing. Just before my turn, I heard the person who was in charge of the audition whisper to another person, pointing at me saying I was a little too fat. After hearing this, I felt embarrassed, insulted, and a bit angry with myself (my body), and then I decided not to go through the audition. I left the audition. Ever since then, I never wanted to go any audition, no matter what. Later years I realized that I was so stupid and so impatient. I should have gone through with it no matter what to experience it. To have various experiences is not a bad thing. I was too self-conscious, too embarrassed, and lacked self-esteem.

    My sister bought a small "Yang Qin" with 30 Chinese Yuan. "Yang Qin" is similar to hammered dulcimer, which is a stringed musical instrument. But a Yang Qin is bigger and has more notes (a broader range of notes). This musical instrument has such a beautiful sound. When my sister left home, she gave it to me. It was such a wonderful gift and also my first step into music. I started to practice by myself without any lessons because, at that time, there were no private instructors to give lessons. Only professional Performance Company offered to its employees. I started practicing scales by hitting the string with a little hammer, then started to play a simple song that I knew, then later practice some other different songs. Some years later, I realized I needed someone's instruction on how to practice correctly and get some technical skills. Through my sister's friend, I found an "instructor" who was not professional but played in a small band in the Tractor Company. I took two private lessons from him. That was helpful. I wrote down his instructions and essential tips, practiced every day. I started to practice more difficult music pieces, even solo pieces. If not happy with my practice, I would practice non-stop until I got it, and the music sounded better. I sometimes practiced two hours at a time; sometimes, I practiced until midnight. I forgot neighbors were sleeping. I was so focused on being a good player. I finally got good at this and played solo in high school with great success. From this, what I found out for myself is: an active person, goal setter, doesn't want to quit, and little bit of OCD can help. Those days the music was all about Mao, the leader of China. All I ever played was this kind of music. Some of the love songs were not allowed to play in those years. Later, when China changed its leader, the situation changed.

During these years, my parents paid very little attention to me; they were dealing with many things that happened during the cultural revolution. I did not learn many personal things from my mother. When I got my first girl thing at age 12, I panicked; I thought I was sick and bleeding needed to see a doctor. It was my sister who told me it was normal for a girl at this age and she told me what to do and no need to panic. At that time, nobody knew what love meant; we did not expect anything either. But we lived with whatever happened, whatever life dished out, we just went along with whatever the situation was, trying to be safe.

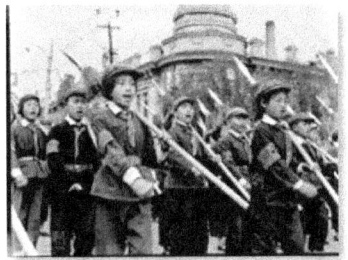 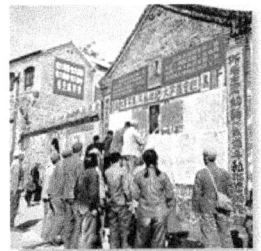

1. Little Red guards join the parade
2. Posters were everywhere

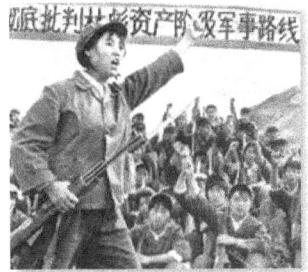 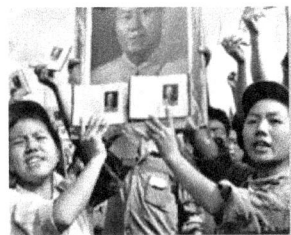

3. Red Guards shouted at government officials
4. Holding Mao's "Red Book."

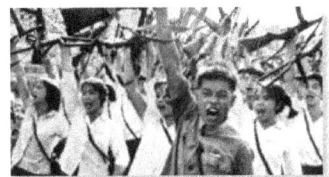 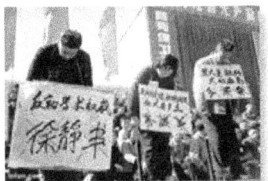

5. Red Guards with guns, protect Chairman Mao.
6. Unfortunate people

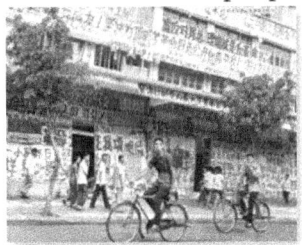 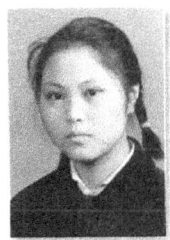

7. Posters were everywhere
8. Me, very confused during the Cultural Revolution

Chapter 3: Moving from City to Town

In 1971, the government officials were still treating my father like he was "being a follower of capitalism" despite all of his hard work and being a long-time loyal member of the Communist party. He could not understand what was going on. He followed communist strategies all the time but was still being treated poorly; he was baffled. For punishment, he was sent to "Five Seven Cadre School (Wu Qi Gan Xiao)" for one year, to be "re-educated." It is a semi-prisoner type of life. He was assigned to do cleaning work, feed pigs, and some farming work. Also, he would go to the daily class to be "re-educated." He was at a loss, did not understand all of this nonsense that he had to go through. My brother and I lived with my mother, who was not happy and cranky all the time. I often thought, "why is my mother so cranky?". Later I realized she carried a lot of stress at that time and had no one she could talk to about it.

In 1972, my father was assigned to work in a Manufacturer of Meters & Apparatus in a small town named Hong Jiang, a mountain area in Hunan Provence. Even though it was still the same province, it was far from the city of Changsha, where we all lived and grew up. There he was assigned as a factory chairman (Shu Ji) in a branch factory. It was a government-owned manufacturer and had over 2000 employees.

In China at that time, the city and town were very different. The city was clean, convenient, organized, civilized, better education, better economic status, better road, and transportation. The town was considered a lower level of "small city" was less clean, less convenient, less organized, less civil, education varied, less money in family, poor road condition and transportation, lower economic status. City people are proud of living in the city, don't want to live in town or farmland, which had such an unfortunate living situation.

Moving to Hong Jiang was upsetting to my mother. She did not want to move to the little town. We all knew this was a punishment from the "government." My father decided to go by himself, knowing that he was going to be very lonely. I loved my father, the most honest person on the planet; I felt terrible not being able to help him. I knew he needed as much emotional support as he could get. On the day before he left for Hong Jang, I wrote him a note, "Dear Father, don't worry too much. You will do well over there. I support you with all my heart." My father was in tears after reading my note. He could not believe that I was the only one in the family who supported him (most of my siblings were not home, left me, and my younger brother). My letter inspired him, and he went to Hong Jang the next day.

After my father left for Hong Jiang, we wrote to each other as often as we could. He told me Hong Jang was a beautiful place with mountains and a river. He said there were so many good things about Hong Jiang. It was cool in the summer (Chang Sha was very hot in summer) and not too cold in the winter. There was lots of fresh fruit. He said you could even pick wild fruit yourself in the mountain, such as kiwi fruit (which tasted five times better than the kiwi fruit we find in the supermarket), berries, and wild plums. He told me that he lived right next to the river and had a lot of fish for dinner. My father, knowing how much I enjoyed eating fish, said we could eat it every day. He said Hong Jiang was less expensive to live. Attracted by the nature of the scene he described, and the fresh fruit which I loved; I wrote to him that I would move to Hong Jang and live with him. I also knew he was very lonely over there, and needed a family.

I decided to convince my younger brother, telling him we could be happier if we moved to Hong Jiang. The reality was not that I wanted to move to Hong Jiang; it was because I missed my father and wanted to support him; I didn't want him to be lonely. My mother had no choice because my brother and I both agreed to move to Hong Jiang. All my older brother and sisters had already left home, and only my younger brother and I remained at home. It was two against one. One year later, my brother and I moved to

Hong Jiang, but my mother did not want to go, so she remained living in Changsha for several years. All of this happened just one year before I graduated from high school.

Transportation to Hong Jiang was only by bus, truck, or car. There were no proper roads at that time. It was a two-day bus trip on the dusty mountain road from Changsha to Hong Jang. Now China has changed so much, it only takes 4 hours driving to Hong Jiang from Change Sha on the highway (if no traffic).

You would not believe the difference between a medium-sized Chinese city and a little town. It's like comparing Brooklyn (NY) today, and a New Hampshire village in 1910! Hong Jiang was a beautiful place nestled in the mountains with a river flowing through it. However, since the town was so poor at that time, the living condition was not pleasant. Each day I had to walk 2.5 miles (4 kilometers) to go to school, rain or shine. The road was either dusty or muddy, depending on the weather. On rainy days, we got mud splashed all over our clothes when a car passed by us. On sunny days, the dust would cover every part of your body after walking home from school. But I could get one delicious kiwi fruit for a penny! That Kiwi fruit is different from the kiwi in a supermarket: Ten times more delicious. With a nickel, I could get a big grapefruit! And more: the Yangmei, beautiful and delicious big berry I bought for just 5 cents a pound! That part I liked.

My school in Hong Jiang was so poor. There was no comparison with the school I had left in the City of Chang Sha. In Chang Sha, I was in the "First School of Changsha," which was one of the best schools for many years in Changsha. In the Frist School of Changsha, we not only studied, but also did some after school activities, such as performing art group, or athletic team, etc. I was part of the music team of the performing art group. I played Yang Qin (Hammered Dulcimer) in the "band." In Hong Jiang, the school I went to is called "First School of Hong Jiang," also a good school. But in Hong Jiang, we were not only required academic study but also required to do physical labor. It included cleaning the classrooms, outside classrooms and lawn, pull the weeds, carry sand

and rocks to school from the river, for some, also construction work on the school. I was never asked to do any physical work except cleaning classrooms in school at Chang Sha. But here in the Hong Jiang school, I had no choice because everyone was doing it. Carrying sand and rocks from the river to school was way too hard for me. The boys were laughing at me because they never saw such a fragile person who could not carry things. I hated this because I never carried any sand in my life. I was a little depressed in the beginning: I did not expect such a big difference, and many of the things were beyond my physical ability. I was not ready for this, and I disappointed myself. But I was happy to stay with my father.

Now when I think back, carrying sand and rocks is not a bad thing, it is a type of physical exercise. It was me who did not see the positive side of things that I wasn't used to it; it was me who was not willing to take challenges, and it was me who could not accept the life as it was. And, it was me who kept the snobby attitude of a city girl. I now realized how many mistakes I had made.

Students in my class were very kind to me, and soon I made friends and then felt more comfortable and more relaxed. The kids knew that I came from a "big City"; they gave me a lot of attention. But I had the attitude of a "proud city girl." I made myself aloof from most students and teachers. Later in life, I regretted having behaved like that way. I know it was not fair. I was too snobby. I guess from the experience of good and bad; I learned a lot about myself. One thing I learned was to be humble.

Since many of the teachers came from the more prominent city schools, the quality of teaching was good even though the school was poor. The teachers went to small towns for many different reasons. My teacher, who also came from a big city, was excellent. I often thought she suffered from depression because I noticed she looked sad some times. I rarely saw her smile, but she was very helpful to all students. Because of having good teachers, my grades were good. I thought her depression might be from relocation to a small town, just like me. I heard that she might be from a wealthy family or an educated family; therefore, she got sent to a small town.

As time went by, I got used to Hong Jiang. I realized that people from Hong Jiang were simple, kind, genuine, sincere, honest. Soon I had many good friends, and they were wonderful! Very often, I ate at my friend's home, where their parents cooked so well. I especially loved their homemade pickles. In summer vacation, I joined the city performing-art team, where I was in the band playing Yang Qin. Our performing art team went to the countryside from village to village to perform singing, dancing, and other entertainment pieces. It was tiring but so much fun. We carried our bedding and instruments; we would walk along the ridge of the fields every day from one place to another; we ate together, sleep in farmer's houses, and had no other worries but to have fun. It was all volunteer work. One month of travel on foot and we played many places. I made friends and had a very different experience with this team.

In February 1974, I graduated from the "First High School" in Hong Jiang. Due to government policy at the time, all graduates had to go to the countryside (farmland). The purpose of this policy was to have young people understand that life should include hard work, and hard work will bring you everything. They called this "Learn to be self-sufficient." This movement affected the whole country, and we, along with others, were called "Educated Urban Youth, who go and work in the countryside or mountain areas."

The Chinese leader Mao Tse Dong came from a farm family. He thought everyone should know where the rice/grain came from and how to be self-sufficient. Chairman Mao believed that all school kids who have reached the age of 16 must eat with farmers, live with the farmers, and labor with the farmers. He believed that by learning to work hard and being self-sufficient, China could become strong.

It was such a big deal sending kids to the country. On February 25, 1974, all the kids were gathered together, carried our bedding and personal belongings to line up in Hong Jiang downtown, waiting for a bus at a big open space. Many people from the City of Hong Jiang, and my father's factory came to see us off; it was like having a big farewell party outdoors. February was still cold, all of us standing outside in the big open space listening to the speeches of the Mayor and other people, all nonsense to me. After these speeches, the buses one by one took us to various farms in different towns and counties. Many other kids and I went to a town called Hui Tong (Huitong) in Hunan Province.

Chapter 4: Memorable Farm Life

If you think the town of Hong Jiang was not so good, the transition to Hui Tong was much worse; if you think carrying sand was too hard, working in the Hui Tong countryside was ten times harder, and it was daily hard work. Nothing could be worse than this.

On the first day we arrived in the countryside, we had no place to stay. Twenty of us had to stay in the attic of the farmer's house with our cotton bedding, no mattress, no heat, no electricity. Our cushioning was made using layers of rice straw. We used an oil lamp, flashlight, and candles for lighting. There were no windows, no walls, but some straw bundled up to make a "wall" on the side of the attic. The cold February wind blew directly through the leaky walls; it was cold, and there was snow outside. We brought some alcohol to drink and made our dinner.

Since we had each brought some food from home, we all shared. While we ate supper, we also joked and drank a lot of liquor (I only drank a little, boys drank a lot more than girls). After dinner, we chatted for a while and told stories and jokes. One kid started to sing a song with a somber melody, but the words described "school kids leaving home, family, and going to the harsh countryside." All of a sudden, one kid started to cry. That was like lighting a fuse, and then everyone began to cry except me. It was an unfortunate situation and very heavy in our hearts. I did not cry not because I was strong; it was because I was confused, puzzled, exhausted, angry, depressed, numb, and maybe melancholy. I could not see any future. I was thinking that if this is my fate, to be in the countryside working as a farmer, I may have to be part of it and accept the bad luck. I felt a deep sense of loss.

It was just the beginning; the hard work was waiting for me! At that time, I did not understand the Dao, change, the stages of life, and the way things go. The situation in China was controlling me, many things were not right, but there were no answers to it. There was no way anyone could make it better. Now I understand why there were so many angry people at that time.

When we got to the countryside, some of us were assigned to build an orange farm in the commune; others assigned to orange farms in different villages. But in the busy seasons, which was in spring (sowing) and fall (harvesting), everyone would go to the village to help the farmers planting rice (Spring) and harvesting rice (Fall).

To build an orange farm from nothing, we had to start from the most basic steps. You can imagine how, when the Pilgrims came to America to start a new life, how they worked was how we worked (maybe we had a little advantage).

At first, we had no place to sleep; then, we got assigned to different farmer's houses. Two or three students were assigned to live with one farmer's family, but we lived in a farmer's shed. We realized right away; we had to build our own living space, our housing. At the request of some students, the government provided some money for the housing project. Since there were no roads to transport building materials to our farm (only two miles away), the boys had to walk miles to bring wood from the forest to our farm. Since there was no road, we had to move building material (wood) by the river. Following the local farmers, the boys tied all the logs together and laid them flat, then put them in the water letting the current carry the logs to a place near our farm, which in China we call "Fangpai." There were no safety measures; early on, a boy named Wang Chunlai was injured when he was pulling the wood out of the water. The boys (about a dozen of them) carried logs on their shoulders from the river to the farm. All the houses in the area were wooden. After all the materials had arrived, the boys, under the guidance of local farmers, began to build our "house": lots of hammering, lifting, shouting, laughing, even singing. All this hard work was unpaid, and nobody complained. I guess we didn't know anything about "getting paid," or we had no choice. We thought this is what life is supposed to be.

The house we needed to build was a long, one-story building that could accommodate 40 people. There are 20 rooms; each room can house two people, we have about 40 people, from different schools and towns. To have a place to cook, we needed to build an outdoor kitchen because it would take too long to make an indoor kitchen, and there was no money for an indoor kitchen, but we needed to eat. Building an outdoor kitchen with manual labor, we first had to carry the bricks to our farm from a place two kilometers away. We used flat bamboo sticks (split bamboo in the middle to make two half sticks, also called carry poles). Each pole had two bamboo baskets attached to the two ends with rope. We placed bricks into the two bamboo baskets, then carried the flat bamboo over our shoulders to transport the blocks. That's how we moved the bricks.

We carried the bricks on our shoulders with a bamboo stick walking more than 1 mile (2 Kilometers) to our place all day long. That was one of the hardest jobs I was ever assigned to do; I hated it! I could not carry so many bricks on my shoulder! Each load weighed about 80 to 100 pounds. With each passing step, the bricks seemed heavier and heavier. On my first trip of carrying the stupid bricks, after walking only less than ½ miles with the yoke (bamboo stick) on my shoulder, I could not walk anymore. I sat down and started to cry. I felt hopeless and unable to move an inch. There was still a long way to go. My shoulders were red, painful, and swollen; my feet had developed blisters; my legs were aching. The 100-pound load of bricks felt like it weighed ten times as much. I was desperately crying for God's help. Or anyone who can help.

One girl named Feng Yue Zhi came back after not seeing me at the main "office." She knew I might have trouble with this kind of work. She took my bricks and carried them to the designated location. I felt like a fool, stupid, weak person, embarrassed, but I forever thank her for helping me carry those bricks. Without her help, I did not know what could have happened. I felt like she saved my life.

I was the worst "farmer," ...and the slowest, especially at digging. Other people can complete the work much faster than me. I was just a city girl who had never done any hard work. The others had already practiced this kind of labor from living in a small town. To them, carrying heavy weights on their shoulders, and digging in the ground were no big deal. They seemed not to have the problems that I was having. To me, this was extremely hard.

So began my country life.

We finally completed the house and were able to live in it. Each room had two roommates, and roommates made food together, washed clothes together, and ate together. At night, all of us got together to enjoy conversation, jokes, telling stories and singing. I enjoyed the group fun, but not hard work because I had never done this kind of work.

We began work on terracing the fields in the hills, digging the dirt to make flat ground for planting and growing orange trees for the future. All the hills needed to be worked to have flat spaces. Every day we dug with shovels and hoes on the hills, moving dirt and rocks, eight hours a day rain or shine. On rainy days we had mud all over our body. Our clothes pasted with mud; on sunny days, our sweat was continually dripping. In the summertime, the temperature sometimes reached 38 C degrees during the day. Our clothes were wet all day long. Our hands quickly became blistered. While very painful in the beginning, calluses developed to protect them later on. Our skin darkened from being exposed to the sunlight all day. Every part of my body ached in the beginning but felt better as the days went on. I became stronger day by day. Several months later, I was able to carry 100 pounds and moving the dirt and rocks like it was nothing. I then realized that a human could get used to anything, like me, such a whiner, became more capable and stronger. But, please don't ask me to do this again.

We terraced the fields during the "off-season," which was between rice planting season and harvest season. In "planting season," we all went back to our division village to help out. From the end of March to the beginning of May, we were ordered to go to the rice fields for several weeks to plant rice sprouts into the cold, muddy, wet fields. That was another hard time of the year. Stepping into the cold, murky, wet fields with bare feet sent chills through one's bones and whole body. We had to gather rice sprouts in a bundle and then plant eight to twelve sprouts into each spot about eight to ten inches apart. All-day, every day, we'd bend over planting one endless field after another. It wasn't just the cold, the mud, or the back-breaking bending all day; the other worst part was having leeches stick to my leg. I was freaking out, seeing leeches on my leg. I'd try to pull it off, but could not. It stuck to my leg so hard like glue. The harder I pulled the leech, the tighter it would bite onto my leg. The farmers then told me that if I hit on my legs violently, the leech would vibrate off. I learn that trick and then was able to get rid of the leeches. The wound from a leech bite left non-stop bleeding. I later learned that the leech bite has a chemical that prevents blood clotting. All of us were frightened and some in tears over the leech bites in the beginning, then later got used to it, especially after the peasants had told us there were no complications from leech bites. I prayed every day for this nightmare to end.

The second busy season is in hot August. Once the rice ripened and turned yellow, we marched back out to the fields to harvest the grain by hand with a sickle, and a simple pedal-driven threshing machine to take the rice off the stems. It went like this; we'd go into the field cut a swath of stems with a knife, shaped like the number seven, then gather the stems into bunches; after that, we used a special machine to remove the grain from the stems. We put the grain in two big round baskets so we could carry them on a pole on our shoulder from the field back to the storage room. Yet another tough time of the year. Imagine it's in August. We would be out in the baking sun for many hours, and we worked eleven hours a day with only a one-hour lunch break. Some people fainted repeatedly; I am sure it was from dehydration. From early morning to late evening, we worked all day long with the farmers. I remember a boy in our group who cut his finger while harvesting the rice plants. He sat on the bank and cried. I almost cried from seeing him, a man crying, coupled with the amount of work we were doing, this was all too much to handle. I kept telling myself: there is no escape, no other way, you have to do it!

During the planting season and harvest season, I stayed in one farmer's home, ate with them, slept in a small room, even had my own "home-made toilet" (dug a hole, then put two wooden boards over it). The farmer's whole family was very kind to me, which made me feel a little better. If I had not been with this family, I might have gone crazy.

Imagine, all this hard work was for free; not a penny was earned. I could not say it was "slavery," but the reality was similar to it.

After harvesting the rice, we'd flood the field again, and replant rice into the field just like we did in springtime. We had two rice-planting seasons. Every spring and late summer, we went back to the rice fields for planting, then harvest again in early winter. The amount of work was unbelievable.

During the offseason, we were asked to do other work, which involved planting sweet potato, corn, vegetables, soybean, cotton, and tending to animals. This was how I learned to do planting work. Planting work was not too hard, but to dig out the pig manure from the pigpen was the most disgusting thing I have ever done. I would never want to do it again in my life.

We were only 17 years old at the time; a few people were a little older. Sometimes we felt very lonely and sad. We were far away from family. We would sometimes walk to the town to go to movies or buy some necessities for daily use. Every Sunday, we went to the farmer's market to get some meat, fruits, vegetables so that we could have one decent meal per week. Once a while we wanted to go home, we would need to walk 1 to 2 hours to town (depending on the road and weather), then take a 2-hour bus ride to Hong Jiang. Every time we went home, the family cooked some meat dish then put it in a big jar so that we could bring it back to the countryside. One jar might last a week if we didn't share too much with others. But most of us id share with others, we knew that none of us had good food. I remember one time we had no vegetables or meat; we cooked hot pepper soup with rice.

We sometimes fought, sometimes argued, sometimes laughed, and sometimes had fun chatting and joking. Sometimes we played musical instruments. We were still young and confused most of the time. We did not date (can you believe that)? All we did was eat, sleep, work, and visit other friends on Sunday. During visiting friends, we always slept over so that we could spend more time chatting. One time I got scabies from sleeping over. I did not know it was scabies, which is highly contagious. So, after visiting another friend, I gave her scabies. During visiting friends, we used their bedding, towel, and anything in a friend's room. The scabies was not easy to treat. There were no real doctors in the countryside, but there were many "Barefoot doctors," who took several months training and then were able to prescribe medication. The barefoot doctor told me that sulfur could cure scabies, but I tried sulfur cream, it did not work. Finally, I had to use sulfur to mix in the water then take a bath with sulfur water. It worked. Later in medical school studying infectious disease, I learned what scabies is and how to prevent it.

I remember sometime in the second year, I felt very down. I thought I was useless, boring; life was dull, and farm work is not my cup of tea. I felt life was such a waste being a farmworker in the countryside after so many years in school. I wanted to be alone, away from anything and anyone. I was very depressed and did not want to interact with other people. I asked the farm leader to be alone working in a pig farm in the valley. I came up with a way to convince the farm leader: "I would like to learn various farm work, such as gain knowledge of feeding pig." I thought if I could work on a pig farm, I could live by myself, and nobody would bother me except do my job. I had no experience with or knowledge about feeding pigs. I didn't know anything about pigs except eating pork.

The farm leader thought it was a good thing that I wanted to learn, and he assigned me to the pig farm where there were nine pigs. He also appointed two older men to assist me with pig food. The two older men were responsible for collecting the pigs' food from particular weeds and grasses, and I was responsible for cooking it and feeding the pigs at regular intervals.

The pig farm was in a remote valley, with no one around within a one-mile radius. Just the three of us lived and worked there. It was tranquil day and night except for hearing the sounds of birds, crickets, and frogs. The two older men (age 60s?) lived in one room, and I lived in another room. There was no electricity, so we used candles or oil lamps and flashlights for lighting at night. The men were out all day gathering the weeds and grasses for me to cook, while I was home preparing the weeds grasses for feeding the pigs. I would then cook meals for the three of us. Sometimes, I had to go out to cut weeds and grass for the pigs. The nine pigs were in six different pens. Some pens had two pigs, and others had only one. I had no idea why the pigs were grouped this way. I could not identify which one was female or male; or how old they were. They were all dirty and ugly looking.

We used stream water for living and cooking. We had to use buckets to take the stream water then use it for any purpose. I didn't communicate much with the two old guys, even though they were very kind to me. We worked separately during the day. At nighttime, we sat around the fireplace and chatted a little bit. Mostly, they told jokes. I sat and laughed. They were always very nice to me, always helping me any time I needed help. Sometimes I would wash their clothes in the stream. Sometimes I would sew buttons for them. We helped each other and felt like a small family.

As time went by, I learned quickly. I felt better in the pig farm: peaceful, calm, soothing, no stress. I started to enjoy my work. I began to smile and laugh and talked more than in the beginning. Maybe I was more at one with nature; perhaps the valley had some healing energy; maybe there was less interaction with many things; maybe I didn't have to overthink things, just simple work, and life;

maybe the pigs; maybe the birds, crickets and frog's singing; maybe the amount of work was not too hard. Who knows what happened? I now think back, and it was pure nature in the valley that nourished and cleansed my soul and body.

One afternoon, I heard some noise then saw a black pig went crazy trying to jump over the fence to the next pen with another pig. It was squealing loudly. I thought the black pig was sick and needed some medical attention or had rabies disease. I was scared and didn't know how to handle this situation. The pig finally jumped over and fought with the white pig in that pen. I ran out and yelled to the two old men and told them that the pigs were fighting. They quickly came to the pig room, thinking something serious had happened. When they saw the black pig grab onto the back of the other pig, they laughed. They laughed so hard while I still had no clue what was going on and why they were laughing. Finally, I realized I was a fool. Several months later, the white mother pig gave birth to 8 little piglets; I assisted in the delivery, helping the old men. It was the first time I learned how the pig babies came out. They were adorable, small, maybe less than a pound, lovely, delicate, and vulnerable. Several months later, I was assigned to go back to the orange field after I got used to the pig farm. I guess the leader thought I had enough experience with the pigs, and the orange field needed more people working.

Upon returning to work at the orange farm, my stress level was much less. I went on with my regular country life.

In my third year of country life, some of us started going back to the city because government companies were hiring, they were short of workers. Some companies went to the countryside to hire students since we had a high school education. We were called "Educated Young Fellows" (Zhi Shi Qing Nian). This was exciting news; it meant we had hope of starting a new career. Usually, each firm would hire 2 to 4 people. We all wished for these jobs. Some firms only hired boys, and some would hire both girls and boys. There was a lot of competition and fighting because everyone wanted to get out of the countryside. I wasn't that excited because I didn't like any of these jobs. But I still would like to get out of farm life. I tried to join an Army troop but was not successful. In the Army, you would have the opportunity to do more and learn more; the benefits in the Army were excellent; at least it was better than the countryside. The commune leader would decide who could go to the Army. It was all about who had a good relationship with the commune leader. I was not very good at keeping up relationships with leaders, but they liked me because they thought they could use my father's help.

I then was on the list of pre-Party members. To be a Party-member, one should do something extraordinary. They call it the "test of the party member." The commune leader wanted to keep me in the countryside and wanted me to be a leader. They wanted to test me to see if I was qualified. Their plan was assigning me to a big project: lead 50 men joining with thousands of others, to make a big reservoir in Hui Tong County. This job was going to be three months (with no pay at all). I was not qualified to do this kind of work: I could not handle hard labor, never managed men, and I did not want any of this. But I felt they wanted me as a hostage so that they could get some benefits from my father, such as hire their people to work in my father's factory. There was nothing I could do.

This decision was upsetting some of the country folk (farmers). They did not think it was wise to have a city girl to manage countrymen. China is a very old country having an ancient tradition that women are always subservient to men. So, I understand why this would be upsetting them. Even though they were upset, some of them still respected me. Most of them had no voice anyway. I went forward. I thought if I did well, maybe they would let me go to the army or college.

In the beginning, I was a little excited. I thought it might not be difficult, and did not expect I could fail. I wanted to be successful so that the leader would like me and then allow me to go to college or military.

We arrived at the reservoir construction site (I think it was either November or December). First, we needed to determine in our sleeping place.

There were big tents in a designated location. Women and men lived in different tents. Each tent held at least 50 people. We all slept in our "sleeping bag" on the floor. Our personal belongings were placed next to our pillow: no locks, no suitcases, just bags. We did not have any money, so we did not worry that things would be stolen. We shared an outdoor bathroom. We washed our face brushed teeth and shared a water hose outdoors, and maybe wash our body once a week in a shower room. Every morning we started to work at 8 AM and back for dinner at 6 PM. There was a two hours period for lunch, and we would eat then take a little nap. My job was not only managing these men but also carrying dirt dug from one place to the place where we were building the dam. We walked all day back and forth to build the dam. Eventually, there would be a reservoir for the county. Later, when I went back to visit friends, they told me that the reservoir was a failure.

The tremendous labor was unbearable. We were required to carry dirt (soil) and stone to the reservoir by walking back and forth all day long. There were thousands of people working in this project doing the same labor. There were no machines or equipment. All work had to be done by our hands, shoulders, and feet. My hands were blistering from shoveling dirt into a bamboo bucket. My feet blistered and bleeding from carrying dirt all day long. My shoulders were swollen and very painful from carrying the dirt. I was exhausted by the end of the day and had to force myself to get up every morning. The pain and aches in my body made me feel like I was an 80-year-old women near death. We had no proper food, all we ate was rice and vegetables, sometimes we had meat. It would be considered a healthy diet if I was doing office work. But for that much physical labor, one must eat well and have enough protein and other high-energy food. I had no problem sleeping because I was so tired and exhausted. I fell asleep as soon as I hit the pillow. I could say I collapsed at night after dinner.

After the first week, I knew I was going to fail. I was sick by about the second week; my body ached, plus I had the flu. I had to stay in the tent for three days. The guys started to laugh at me and asked to change leader. I was ready to quit too.

On the 2nd or 3rd week I found out that schools were doing enrollment, I expressed to the commune leaders (commune official) that I would like to go to school (college and university). They rejected me. I guess they did not like that I failed the test they gave me for becoming party member. With tremendous despair and sadness, I did not want to continue to lead and do the hard work anymore. I told the leader I was not able to go on. Not even halfway done, I failed the test.

I returned to the farm before the reservoir was done. I was very fragile, mentally, emotionally, and physically. I felt broken. I felt hopeless, just like being trapped in a dark well and not able to escape, even screaming for help. I walked in the little path and cried and cried. I suddenly stopped and stared at a big tree. I then wished I had a rope with me so I could finish this endless miserable life. But I did not have anything I could use.

I could not go back to my place, so I decided to visited my friend Zeng Jian Ying in a different village. She did not know how much I had been through, how fragile I was, how depressed I was. She knew I was tired, and she washed my clothes, cooked for me, and made me comfortable. My other friends She Jiang Kang, Wang Ming Qi, Kuang Jiang Hua all treated me like I was a victorious soldier returning from battle. They were just happy to see me coming back. I wanted to cry. This was one of my hardest times in the countryside. I needed so much: compassion, mental support, and physical help, anything that would comfort me. I wished somebody would hug me tight and listen to my stories and complaints and share feelings with me, then tell me I'm going to be okay.

I was so determined to get out of this place, I then contacted my sister (she was in charge a Performing Art Company), I asked my sister to help me to get out of there. She then sent two people to our commune, to negotiate with the Commune official and give the reason that they needed me for a leading actress of a special show. The official rejected them again. Once again, I felt extremely hopeless, tired, and angry with these officials. I cried and felt extremely depressed still. I asked myself why life was so hard, why God didn't help me, why other people seemed fine except me, why I had so many difficulties one after the other.

At the beginning of the 4th year, when I was 21 years old, the leaders decided to put me in the elementary school to teach first and second graders. I finally had a little physical break. Teaching was a much better sort of work for me. First, I was able to use my knowledge; second, I always liked to work with children because they are so cute and fun. I enjoyed teaching and had a good relationship with my "children" (students). I not only taught them but also would play games with them. The kids liked me very much. I taught math, language, art, and physical education. I repaired their clothes if I saw they were ripped and sewed on their buttons. If any child got sick, I gave them my medication (I brought from home), or let the kid stay with me until they felt better. The parents (farmers) were very emotionally affected by my care for their children. Many times, they brought food for me to show their appreciation for caring for their children. In China, good food was a big thing (gift) at that time. During my years of teaching in elementary school in the countryside, I felt better because I felt more useful and helpful. Their parents appreciated everything that I did. But I still wanted to go back to the city. I still wanted to go to school. So, my depression was still there.

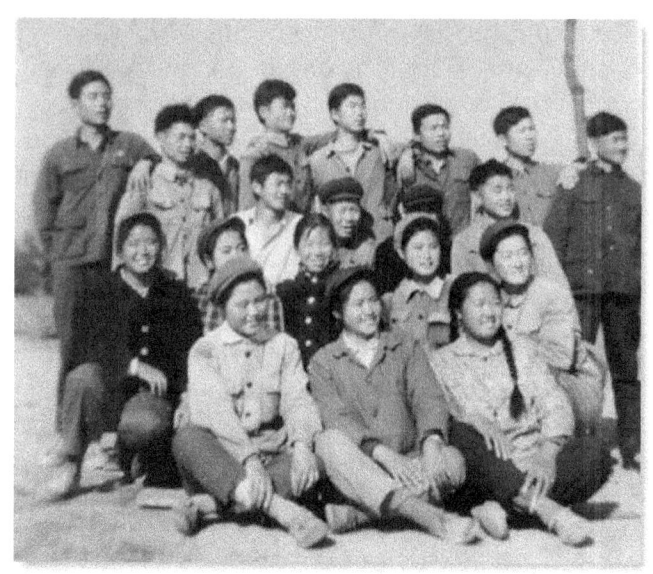

1. Working on the farm

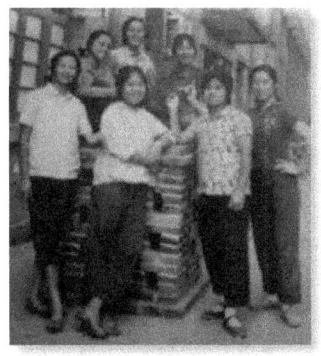 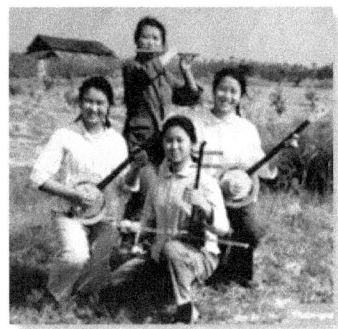

1. Girls visiting downtown Huitong
2. Playing Chinese musical instruments on the farm

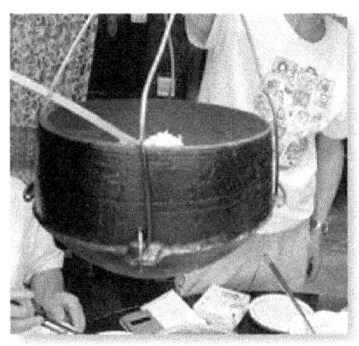 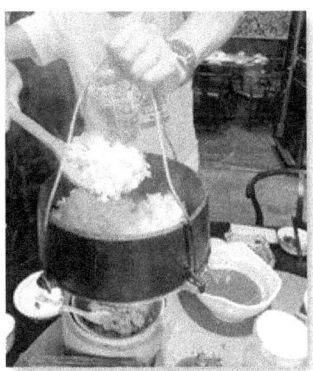

3. Iron rice cooker pot
4. Serving rice cooked over a wood fire.

Chapter 5: Easier Farm Life

When I was teaching in the country school, I lived above the classroom on the second floor. There were two rooms on the second floor; I used one. A male teacher was staying in the room across from mine.

He had a reputation for being a "weird man." Everyone told me he was an orphan. I also heard that he went to prison for several years, but I did not know why. They warned me to be careful. In China, you would be treated as an enemy if you went to prison for whatever reason. Just the two of us lived in this building. He was ten years older than me, and he rarely smiled. Everyone said he was strange, always got angry for every little thing. I didn't seem to have a problem with him except for being a bit afraid of him. Anyway, he was nice to me.

He was an excellent cook and always brought food to me. Sometimes he asked me to join him for dinner. He wasn't shy but rather demanding. Sometimes he asked me to fix his clothes and buttons; other times, he did not talk much. In the wintertime, there was no heat in the room. On snowy days, he would bring a blanket to me, knowing that my bedding was too thin. He sometimes offered to let me go his room to share the "charcoal heat box" in his room. (I didn't have any heat). When there was ever some conflict, he always took my side and helped me to get out of the situation. Sometimes he yelled at other people just for me. He never touched me nor kissed me. He did not even shake hands when we first met. But he treated me like a baby sister. I felt like he was a big brother. I felt good because I felt like I was protected and cared for all the time. Maybe that was what I needed at that most challenging time of my life in the countryside. Later, I missed him; I missed him even after graduating from medical school and working in the hospital.

As the days went by, our relationship got easier. We felt more comfortable with each other, and I wasn't afraid of this man anymore. One day, I was curious. I asked him about his girlfriend. (I had heard that he had a girlfriend before). Surprisingly, he became furious. He became so angry with me for asking this question, he shouted at me and was very upset. He was a completely different person. He asked me never to mention this again. I was so scared because this was the first time he was mad at me. I was almost in tears and promised him never to mention it again. He then realized he should not frighten me, but he did not talk much for a while. Several days later, he was calmer, and he told me the story: He and his girlfriend were both leaders in the "Red Guard" during the Cultural Revolution. He was a commander of this Red Gard group. As we know at that time, China was in chaos, Red guard groups fighting with each other. He and his girlfriend loved each other and did everything together. She followed him everywhere, assisted him with Red Guard commanding work. She swore that she would stay with him no matter what happened, they were so much in love. Just before the end of the Cultural Revolution, he was accused of being a "Counter-Revolutionary" and sentenced to jail for five years. After he went to prison, his girlfriend left him and never even visited him. They never saw each other after that. His heart was broken. He felt cheated, played, manipulated, betrayed. His love for her was so deep, almost like a story in a movie. Ever since, he became quiet, weird, strange, tried to avoid any conversation about her; and he didn't talk to others much either. He tried to forget this sad story and painful experience. I was almost in tears after I heard his story, I sympathized with him. I felt terrible about asking this and having brought back his unhappy memories. In China, these kinds of things often happen due to political pressures. But he was so in love with her and did not expect that she could leave. After this incident, I learned to be careful not to say anything unless it was related to teaching. I also showed more kindness and more care to him. I tried to do more for him, even washed his clothes. Sometimes I tried to cook for him. I just felt he had nobody in this world but me. But we were not dating at all, just friends.

This relationship was a little strange. We both felt very close but not in love. It might have been just because we needed each other during the hard life in the countryside. We never touched each other, never hugged, never kissed, never talked about any personal or emotional things. Even though I was mature enough to date, I would still only love him as a very close friend. Besides, he was too old for me (he was ten years older than me). Many years later, I often thought about him. I missed him as a big brother, protector, and good friend. I felt safe when he was around. I missed having this kind of man in my life.

In 1983, when I was working in the Huai Hua District Hospital, he came to see me and told me that he got married. As usual, he brought me some food. I was so happy to know that he had found someone to share his life with. But I still miss him. Many years later, I heard that he died from cancer. I felt very sad about losing my best male friend.

Country life was tough, not just a dull life and hard work. The hardest thing was mental exhaustion and hopelessness, no guidance, and a feeling there was no future. It felt like I was sitting in the darkness and would never see the light. I continued to have a confused mind, at a loss, no direction, no books to read, no activities besides visiting other friends in the countryside in different villages. Especially after seeing some of my friends were hired and left for jobs in the city, the loneliness became more intense. I felt it was such a waste that I could not use my talent, could not find joy anywhere in life. And the worst part was, I had no one to share my feelings with, but I just had to swallow them down. I did not talk to my family because they were all strictly following the orders and did whatever the government said; nor could I share with my friends because they experienced the same thing. Maybe this is why I so valued my one male friend, who I could trust, rely on, and feel safe with, at least.

I was teaching in elementary school but was working for free. I did not get paid for this job. But it was much better than working in the mud fields, easier on the body, and it was much cleaner. I was happy, but I did not have money. Families gave me 10 yuan (USD 1.50) a month, but that was hardly enough. I then found a way: sell some of my clothes and shoes to some of the farmers, 2 yuan for each shirt, 2 yuan for a pair of shoes. They were happy to get cheap clothes and shoes, and I was glad to get some money to buy meat, vegetables, and snacks. And a bus ticket. We did not need much, but these were necessities.

Farmers liked me a lot. I always brought them some medicine every time I went back home. I took some medicine from my parents. I sometimes gave the farmers some of my clothes and other souvenirs if I went to town and went shopping.

In 1977, the leader in China changed. Deng Xiao Ping became the Chairman (Mao Zhe Dong passed away in September 1976). Deng was instrumental in building a better economy in China. He initiated many big projects and economic reforms in China. He ended many of "Mao's rules." One of which was: "only party members can go to college or university." He made a public announcement that whoever can pass the college entrance examination would qualify to go to school. That was like a bomb that shook every student, including myself, to their core. I was so happy and excited to hear this. I started to see the possibility of a bright future. My heartbeat grew faster every day, and I started singing again. I was so excited. I was going to take the National Pre-College Test. After four years of country life without touching a book, I had to borrow high school books from many different sources. For several months I had to study very hard to prepare for this particular test. Since it meant so much to me, I had to give up everything but study. I taught during the day and studied at night until 1 AM every single day. Sometimes students came upstairs to wake me up in the morning.

At that time, I didn't care about anything else. I just wanted to pass the test, get out the country life, and go to school. When I filled out the form that indicates the choice of school, I put down "Medical School" as my first choice. I always wanted to help sick people, especially after country life, where I saw so many illnesses.

My second choice was the "Railroad Academy" because I always liked to travel. My third choice was "Postal/Telecommunication." Many of us were preparing for the test. I felt like the whole country was preparing for the test. I was facing a big challenge.

In November 1977, I received notice that I was enrolled in Hunan Medical University ("Hunan Medical College" at that time), which was founded by Yale University in 1914. It is one of the best Medical schools in China. Upon receiving the note, tears were pouring down my face; my heart was beating so fast, I was shocked by this news. I could not believe my eyes. I couldn't imagine my dream had come true. I finally realized that the hard work was no longer going to burden me, and my future would soon be so promising; my life was going to change for the better. I was determined to study hard and to work hard and be the best doctor I could be.

Farm life, in the end, I feel, was not a bad experience. I learned to be stronger, to be patient, I learned to sow or plant, to build my own projects, learned to raise chickens, to fix my own clothes and shoes, to cook, to be passionate, to take care of myself, to develop and cherish friendships, and so many other things. I became who I am. I now really understand the Dao, the way, the changes in life.

Chapter 6: Busy Life in Medical School

I went to medical school to become a doctor. I saw a lot of sickness when I was working in the countryside. I sometimes took medication from my parents and brought it to the farmers when I saw them suffering from illness. For example, I saw a farmer who had an infection on his leg that never healed; I took antibiotics from my parents and gave them to the farmer. I saw some farmers so skinny, some were malnourished, and others with medical issues. I took vitamins from my parents and gave them to the farmers. I think that was one of the reasons why I choose to go to medical school.

At that time, the Medical school in China was not comfortable. The living conditions for students was perhaps like the US 100 years ago.

In my first year of medical school, I was so excited in the beginning. I felt so good to be able to get out of the hard country life and go to the school I had been dreaming of. I remember saying to my friends, "I will either become a doctor or marry a doctor." But I prefer to be a doctor because I love to help people. There I was, soon to become a doctor. Shortly after, I started to feel the pressure. In China, all the schools have many examinations throughout the year. Chinese schools evaluate students by looking at who gets higher scores on the exams. So, the pressure on students was very high because we did not want to fail. I felt like we studied not to become a doctor but for the test score. I didn't want to fail, so I started to pressure myself. We had 5 to 7 classes per day. After class, we had to spend another 5 hours reviewing the material and trying to memorize whatever we had studied. In medical school, most subjects require remembering: the names of the muscles, bones, name of nerves, cells, biochemical compounds, and how these all work, etc.

There were 500 to 600 students in our grade. 90% of the students studied Medicine, and 10% studied Public Health. My major was Medicine. We all lived in the school dorm, with 4 to 11 people per dorm room. We got up at 6 AM every day. From 6 AM to 7 AM was exercise time. Students first did group exercises, then had a choice of doing various exercises individually. We had breakfast at 7 AM, then went to class at 8 AM. From 8 AM to 5 PM, we were in class (all different classrooms, sometimes in a lab). After dinner, we also would go to the classroom, or sometimes to the library to review the coursework that we learned during classes. Since there were 500 to 600 students all needing to do evening study and there not enough seats and classrooms to accommodate all of us, we had to ask some of our classmates to skip dinner to hold a seat for us, and we would then bring her dinner later when we got there. The classrooms would close at 10 PM, when all the facilities closed, such as library, laboratory, etc. After that, some students came back to the dorm to continue their studies until midnight, sometimes even later.

The lights in the dorm went off at 11 PM because the school wanted students to have a good sleep, as well as to save electricity. The administration controlled the overhead lights, but the outlets were still working. My brother got me an extension cord and a small lamp so that I could plug into an outlet to get light. This way, I could continue to read in bed. Many other students did the same thing. One or two weeks later, a school official found out, and they sent workers to our dorm during class time when no one was there. They took all the extension cords and lamps away. So, that did not work. Some students did not want to quit, and they went outside under the street light to continue their studies. Imagine, reading a book under a streetlight, how many of us can do this? If students knew the teacher, they would be able to use the teacher's office to study. Others had to find different places to get those extra hours of study. We sometimes even used flashlights.

We only had Sunday off. Even with just one day off per week, we still had to read some study material and tried to memorize the coursework. If we went out, we brought books with us to read at the bus stop while we were waiting for the bus and on the bus. If we visit family or friends, we tried to squeeze in some time for reading a book. There was just too much work, and we didn't want to waste any time. We rarely had any party time during those five years. But sometimes our whole class would go to the park to play some group games.

There was only one TV in the whole building on the second floor, controlled by a manager who was in charge of our dorm. Students who had good memory were able to watch TV in the hallway; others couldn't afford to waste time to watch TV. My memory wasn't good, so if I watched TV, I would have to spend extra time to study. That would be my payback.

Since the pressure was so high, one student could not handle the stress, and he attempted suicide. He took a whole bottle of sleeping pills at night and did not wake up until we came back from the class the next afternoon. He was taken to the ER immediately. He lived, but the school discharged him for this kind of behavior. I knew that was not right, but it could not be helped. There was no such thing as a "school counselor" or "guidance counselor." Whatever problem we had, we had to deal with it by ourselves. The bright side was, we became reliable and smarter.

We did not have real a shower or bath facility, but just a "bathhouse." Male students used one side, and female students used the other side of the bathhouse. There was a two-hour period when we could get hot water to bathe. If we missed this two-hour hot water period, we had to take a cold bath. The bath was not like the bath you think of nowadays. Our bath involved using a bucket (holding about two gallons of water) to get hot water from outside of the bathhouse, then carry the bucket to the bathroom. We bathed our body with a wet towel one stroke at a time before soap and after soap, then pour the rest of the water over our body. You can imagine in the wintertime if we missed the two-hour hot water time, washing the body with cold water was like torture. But at that time, we had no choice; we thought this kind of torture was typical.

During the first two years, we ate three meals a day in a big dining hall, eight people per table. There was one rice dish in a big bowl, one vegetable dish in a big bowl, and some other food. We had to divide the food into eight individual portions to put into our bowls. Two times a week, we would have a meat dish. We were not happy with our breakfast of soup, rice, and pickled tofu. Therefore, our class (class 8) wrote a large poster to school officials, asking the school to provide us with steamed dumplings (Man Tou) and porridge for breakfast. It worked! We got dumplings for breakfast.

The first year of school, we were assigned to dig a trench to prepare for war or other crises. I remember it was summer when we were digging, it was sweltering, and we had to have a break. I ate four ice pops to cool myself off. Later I had severe stomach pain and diarrhea. One time we were taking a break from digging, one boy named Li, Chang Gang was still in the trench. I called him loudly, "come up, Li, Chang Gang, take a break." He then came up. Right after he came up, the trench collapsed. You can imagine if he did not come out, he might have been killed by the collapse. He always told me that I saved his life whenever we met during my later trips to China.

During our first or second year, 90% of the students got hepatitis. Most got Hepatitis A, some B. I got Hepatitis A. We all got blood tests. I believe it was from the food we ate (bulk meals). All of us got one pound of sugar that was supposed to "help the liver." During the Hepatitis epidemic in school, the school cut back on courses by removing two courses: Latin and Politics.

One year our school had an athletic event, the boys in our class (class 8) got first place. But the girls in our class got nothing. Ever since then, the boys became famous in the school. The other class (class 7), the girls got first place, the boys got nothing. The girls in class 7 became famous.

Occasionally the school had an outdoor movie. There were so many people and not enough room for everyone to sit in front. So, we had to watch the movie on the back of the screen. At least we got to see the film.

During the school year, I was weak and often got sick. I had chronic bronchitis (non-stop coughing) and was taking antibiotics on and off all year round. I had severe headaches and insomnia. In my fourth year, my insomnia was so bad I got only 2 or 3 hours of sleep each day. Plus, with all the intensive study during the day, I had anxiety. Maybe there were still some old unhappy memories that I was holding onto; cultural revolution, my father's mistreatment, relocation, farm life, etc. I felt weak. I had no strength; my Qi was low and poor. I kept telling myself it will be over soon, but it seemed such a long school year. I now understand why I was weak and often sick: my genes were poor, sitting all day with no exercise, no proper nutrition, no emotional support, studying too hard with no life balance.

We always had meals together. We had a meat dish only twice a week, every Tuesday and Friday. Our anatomy classes were also on Tuesday and Friday. Imagine you just got out of a class working on a cadaver, the same color as our meat dish at lunchtime, how much appetite would you have? Some students even threw up looking at the meat on the table: they looked the same. I had to force myself to eat because this was my only chance to have food with protein. Otherwise, I would be hungry in the middle of the class. It is not allowed to have a snack during the class.

The fifth year focused on practical learning, and students got assigned to hospitals in different cities and towns but in the same Province. When I was working in the pediatric unit (department), I once had to take care of a 5-year-old boy who had kidney disease "Nephrotic Syndrome." The treatment involved using steroids, and it affected his body, face, and immune system. But he had such good spirit and joy; it broke my heart to see him going through this. I was sad but compassionate. I wanted to take him home to take care of him; I wanted to help this boy. Ever since then, I had thoughts of becoming a pediatrician.

The school had a rule that students were not allowed to date, even though aged from 18 to 30. The school wanted us to focus on study, and dating may distract from our study. In some ways, the school was right in other ways it was not. Some students would date secretly, but most students just complied. I was one who complied, but I wished there was no such ridiculous rule. I had a date only one month before graduating from school, and I was 26. One year later, I married that boy, had my first baby one year after marriage. The policy for marriage in China at the time was men had to be age 28, and women had to be age 25. Most people followed this "standard"; others may secretly be "off the standard."

Thinking back, if someone had given me some guidance, taught me how to look for a positive way to balance the negatives, how to search for inner peace, how to let go, how to live with the Dao, I could have avoided a lot of this emotional turbulence. The bright side was: with all the ups and downs, I learned how to figure out things for myself, I become wiser and more capable of doing things.

Chapter 7: Practicing Medicine

In 1982, we were required to join in the national examination for all the Medical schools in China. Our school achieved the top level on the national test. This type of government testing was intended to find out which Medical schools in China had the best teaching quality.

I graduated from medical school in December of 1982. I was assigned to a district hospital in Hunan province after I graduated. I wanted to be a pediatrician because I love children. But the hospital at that time needed an OB-GYN doctor, so the hospital leader asked me to join the OB-GYN team. I had no choice. In China, at that time, the best way forward was to do what the hospital official suggested.

To be an OB-GYN (Obstetrics-Gynecology) doctor was not easy. In my resident years, I worked 12-14 hours a day and often had to get up in the middle of the night to assist surgery. Having just graduated from school, I felt like I knew so little about patient care. We, graduates, absolutely had no clinical experience. That was the reason that we had to put in so many hours working in the hospital for a low salary with hard work. But that was the only way we could gain more experience. I got yelled at some times by the experienced doctors for being either careless or not doing a good job. I knew this was a part of the training, part of the learning that every new, young doctor had to go through. Practicing medicine is not a relaxed job; doctors must be able to handle the pressure; otherwise, do something else. We must be able to take criticism and try to improve our skills as much as we can. Once I realized this, I was able to learn and improve myself faster.

I didn't mind working hard as a doctor, but I didn't like the risk involved with this occupation. There were politics involved with the GYN part. Many times, the doctor had no choice in matters. For the birth control part, all the doctors had to do, as the government required. If you would try to resist or against the government rules or refused to do the work, you might be fired or even go to jail. I didn't like this part, as there was no other choice but to obey. I thought the birth control should be the woman's choice not forced.

The good part of being an OB-GYN physician was we got to see many newborn babies. They were so cute and lovely. We always got candy and red eggs from the mothers who had babies. Sometimes the mother gave each of us a gift and thanked us for doing a good job. The GYN patient even thanked us more for curing their illness. Their way of saying thanks was always giving either a gift or food. But the other downside of this job was the high risk of an accident or something unexpected happening. I didn't personally come across any serious problems, but I saw one doctor who had a sudden incident of losing a pregnant mother in 1987. The bleeding would not stop after she gave birth; at the same time, there was a power failure in the hospital. You can imagine how chaotic the situation was. The baby was saved, but the hospital had to pay a lot to the deceased woman's family to avoid a lawsuit. That sort of thing was rare, but it could happen. When it happens, the patient's chance of survival is low. Now things have improved, and hospitals are well equipped with high technology and new tests to find out early if there are any abnormal situations.

In August 1984, I moved to Chang Sha and worked in a clinic in a manufacturing factory where my husband worked. I was in my eight months of pregnancy.

The factory was small, with only 400 people, and the clinic had two doctors, me and Dr. Tang. This was an easy job compared to working in the hospital OB/GYN department. Dr. Tang and I got along very well. We were like primary care physicians, super easy job doing nothing but prescribing and dispensing medicine to workers who had minor sicknesses. If too severe, we requested an ambulance take the patient to the hospital.

One experience I had in the clinic was risky and that I will never do again.

One day I was by myself, and Dr. Tang was on vacation. It was a sunny and quiet day. I was drinking my tea while organizing the medications, and suddenly a man came into my clinic holding the arm of a woman who was just about to give birth to a baby. She had frequent contractions, and her water had broken. I had practiced as an OB/GYN before, and I had delivered many babies in the hospital. But this time was different: not in the hospital, no help, no medical equipment, and no appropriate bed for delivery of a baby. An urgent case, but the hospital was a one-hour car ride away. With no other choice, I decided to deliver this baby by myself. With the knowledge and skills I had, I kept a calm, steady pace, and asked her husband to help me with certain things. I was a little nervous, and I was sweating, my heart was in my throat. This was because I knew that anything could happen in OB work, such as severe bleeding, stillbirth, breach, baby breathing problem, etc. If something happens, my reputation would be ruined. I kept reminding myself: this is the only choice; otherwise, she could die if delayed.

I reminded myself: I am well trained, I am capable, I have experience, and I will get this baby out safely. Finally, the baby comes out, a beautiful boy with a loud cry. I cut the cord and waited for the placenta to come out. She had a reasonable amount of bleeding. Both mother and baby were safe, and everyone was happy. I almost cried; the danger was over. They wanted to go home right away. I kept her for one hour or so, then gave her some instruction for home care before letting her go. After they left, I was exhausted from the stress. I did it all by myself. Believe it or not, I charged them for the delivery service: 100 yuan, which equals about 14 USD

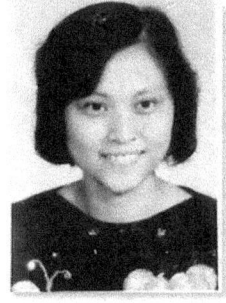 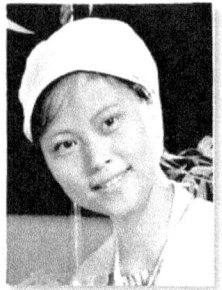

1, 2. First and second year in medical school, so excited!

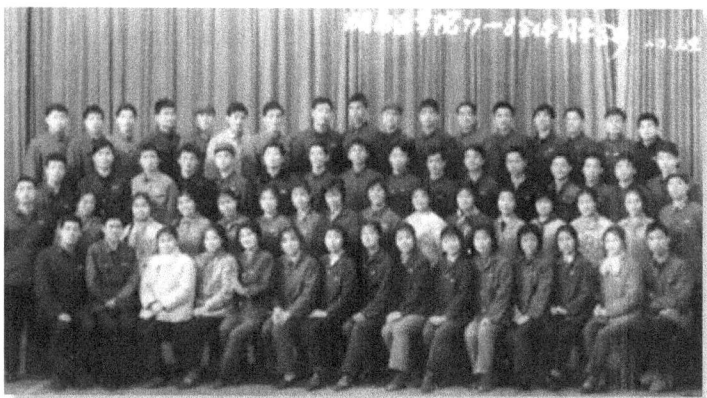

3. My third year in Medical School in 1980,
   I am in the second row, second from right.

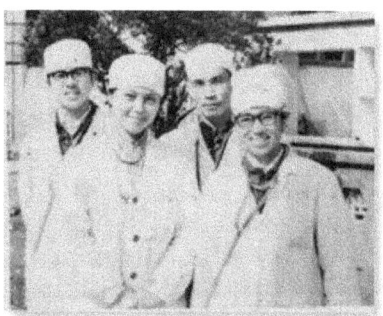 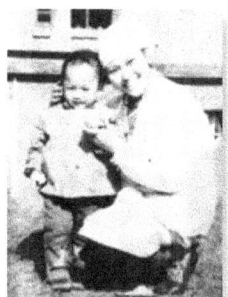

4. Internship in Hongjiang District Hospital
5. Fourth-year medical school, 1981, 1982

Chapter 8: The Pursuit of Love

When I was about 15 or 16 years old, we (when friends were together) used to talk about the ideal (perfect) boyfriend. Most of my girlfriends had a standard model of a boyfriend, which was also the model of "standard boyfriend in China" at that time. It was the idea of: "five yuan." 1. He looks like "yian yuan" (a movie actor). 2. Physical body stature like "yun dong yuan" (athlete). 3. Cooks like "cuei shi yuan" (chef). 4. Sounds like "guang buo yuan" (radio announcer.) 5. His salary must be "yi bai yuan" (100 yuan: Chinese money). At that time, people in China only made between 30 to 50 yuan per month. We were always teasing each other whenever we saw a boy walk by on the street; we would analyze each boy we saw, always finding some "yuan" missing. We had a lot of fun with this joke. But we all knew it was impossible to find all "five yuan" (perfect partner).

Regarding finding love and marriage, the old Chinese culture was very much into having: "family match," "educational match," "height match," "looks match," "money match," etc. Both families should be at about the same level. For example, if your father is a professor, your girlfriend's or boyfriend's father should be at the same level: their parents should be a teacher, cadre, doctor, or professor. It would be less acceptable if your mother or father were a professor, and your boyfriend's or girlfriend's parents were factory workers or farmers. If you have a college degree, your girlfriend or boyfriend should have the same degree or at least close. Otherwise, people would always talk about your personal life behind your back. They would think you are unable to find someone of the same level. Since this tradition has been in China for thousands of years, people got used to it, no matter whether you like it or not. I have seen so many unhappy marriages even after they had the "match." This kind of match ignored the most important issue: true love.

I was always a little rebellious against the rules if the rules did not make sense. I did not think the family match was a good idea. I did not believe money was important. I did not believe perfect looks were important. But I did feel the same education level was necessary, I felt this allowed for a connection of intellect, and with it, you can communicate with each other easily, and understand each other. I learned how important this was much later in life, especially after studying the Dao.

I always had my picture of the perfect boyfriend: a person who knows how to love, a person who understands what true love is, one who knows how to cherish love and how to nurture love just like you fertilize and care for a garden. I wanted to have someone who could understand my feelings, my emotions, and my beliefs. I wanted someone patient who would forgive me if I said something wrong or did something wrong. I wanted someone who would support me, encourage me, and calm me when I was feeling down. I wanted someone with me, to solve problems together, deal with stress together. I wanted someone who understood that it is essential to support each other, help each other, comfort each other, and do things together.

We all know if we fertilize, care for, and water flowers or plants, they bloom beautifully and grow healthy. With your perfect lover, you must nurture your love, and make the romance to last forever.

I always feel the word love has a deep meaning. It is not just finding a boyfriend or girlfriend, and then getting married, or sharing a room or house, and sharing money. It is sharing love, soul, and thoughts, ideas and opinions, feelings, friendship, laughter, pain, and the journey of life. It's sharing everything! It involves honesty, trust, caring, and helping each other, listening, and supporting each other throughout life. True love is thinking about the other person more than yourself. It also involves sacrifice and giving to each other. For anyone selfish, love can never last.

I did not date until I was 26. It was not that I did not want to date; it was because I wished to find the right person. If I had to live with this person for a lifetime, I wanted to find the right man no matter how long I had to wait. If I could not find the right person, I would rather live by myself. Maybe I was a little naïve, or maybe I was living in a fantasy, or perhaps I was a pure spirit (not being practical), or maybe I was too rigid. Now looking back, I think I had 100% good intention but was lacking an understanding of reality.

During the "Cultural Revolution," a brilliant couple accused of being "counter-revolutionary," was sent to the countryside for punishment. Many people were sent to the countryside for this reason (as was my father). At that time, they had nothing but each other. The political pressure was so high, and they lost their freedom. People watched them for any little misstep or action. They had to be very careful with any of their moves and behavior. All their activities were reported to the communist party committee, and people were watching them every minute. The wife was very sick due to lack of nutrition, mental trauma and exhaustion, poor hygiene, and an unhealthy environment; the husband took care of her every single day on the top of doing country labor work. He held her every day, gave her comfort, cooked herbs for her, told jokes, and kept a good sense of humor. He convinced her that one day, their freedom would come, he told her they were going to have children, and the darkness was temporary and would be over soon. Many years later, when the "Cultural Revolution" was over, they were out of country life. They both found good jobs and started a new life again. With the strength of love, they survived all the horror.

This story made me cry. It is carved into my heart and will never go away. We don't have to have everything in our life. But if we have true love, it makes up for many things.

We may or may not find true love. But if our intention is there, and our heart is pure and kind, we will have true love. The amount of work we put into something will always determine the outcome.

Chapter 9: Unfortunate Life

To write this chapter was not easy. I had cried while writing some parts. But it was a huge part of my life, and hopefully, it will have meaning for other people.

I got married when I was 27, and one year later, we had our daughter. My husband, Du Gang, and I knew each other since childhood. Our parents were friends in military college. He was very intelligent, and his memory was incredibly strong. I often asked him to remind me if I needed to do something. I always joked he had a computer brain. Du Gong was quiet, observant, handsome, and very handy. He was very good with electronics. He could even build a TV or radio from scratch.

Life sometimes plays tricks on us. It was a hectic time for me with caring for my daughter, working in the hospital, and being a wife. On October 1, 1987, when our daughter was 3, tragedy struck our family.

I was working in the hospital; my husband said he had a bad headache. I took him to the hospital, where the doctor gave him some pain medication, which only helped him temporarily. Then they gave him some stronger medication for pain. The next morning when he woke up, the headache became more severe, he felt nauseous and vomited. I realized that this wasn't a usual headache; it was much more serious. I took him to the hospital, where I was working at that time. The internist immediately performed a spinal tap, and they admitted him into the hospital because the spinal tap showed blood in his spinal fluid. He was diagnosed with a "Subarachnoid Hemorrhage," which was one of the arteries in the brain bleeding caused by a genetic deformity. During the week that he was in the hospital, he received conventional treatment

(Western). The symptoms would come and go, which meant the situation was still difficult. Doctors suggested that surgery was necessary.

I then transferred him to a bigger hospital, which had the best reputation for neuro-surgery in our province, a teaching hospital of the medical school where I had studied. The doctor in charge of the case was my classmate at Medical School, Dr. Yang. She did standard care, and my husband's symptoms were almost stable. Dr. Yang told me that once he was more stable, he will need surgery. During his stay in the hospital, I visited him every day after work. If I worked a night shift, I would visit him in the morning then go home to sleep after. I did not sleep much worrying about him and my daughter, and working fulltime, and visiting him daily. Every time I visited him, I brought food he liked and told him about our daughter's activities, which made him feel there was no need to worry. He was very moved and said that he would take me to travel to every place in China when he got out of the hospital. I knew he was very much appreciative of my tireless care.

The situation changed drastically one day before the surgery. One morning about 4 or 5 days after being admitted to the hospital, around 8 AM, a young doctor brought in a group of medical students into my husband's room to ask him to explain how his illness started. My husband was in a teaching hospital, where it was not uncommon to have medical students involved in severe cases so that they could learn. The young doctor forgot that my husband was under a type of intensive care that patients should not be startled, excited, or be interrupted during their quiet time. I guess this young doctor forgot his training or was careless. This physician suddenly woke my husband up and started to ask him questions related to his symptoms. He suddenly woke up, then tried to explain the day he had a headache. Within two minutes, my husband started to have a seizure. Shortly afterward, he lost consciences and lapsed into a coma. The hospital did not do surgery, just used medication to control the bleeding in the brain. He remained in a coma for one month. Since this hospital is part of the medical school where I studied, I could not say much, nor did I have the guts to sue the hospital. But I wondered about the quality of the hospital and did not want to go there anymore.

Patients, who have suffered a ruptured cerebral aneurysm, have a period where the body attempts to heal itself by forming a blood clot at that area of the weakened vessel. At the time of the initial bleeding, the patient will experience symptoms such as the "worst headache that they have ever had." After this point, there is a 7 to 10-day "window" when surgery can be performed before the aneurysm may again rupture. During this time, the patient is placed on what is known as "aneurysm precaution." Some of which I previously mentioned. This precaution can also include a dark room, seizure precautions, and other precautions. What occurred with my husband was that he was suddenly awakened from a deep sleep. This sudden excitement caused an increase in adrenaline and resulting high blood flow to the brain. The weakened blood vessel area was unable to handle this powerful increase in the volume of blood, causing it to rupture again. This time he wasn't as lucky as before. The damage was too severe.

He passed away in Nov.19, 1987, at the age of 31, when my daughter was only three years old. He died from the effects of a ruptured cerebral aneurysm due to sudden stirring by the ignorant doctor. We did not get a chance to say good-bye.

That was a tough year for me, physically, mentally, financially, and spiritually. I was 31 years old. The winter was so dark, so cold, and so long. December was tough, and I got sick often. It was one problem after another. Physically I felt fragile. I had bronchitis; then it turned into pneumonia. I had insomnia, headache, and other things. My energy level was very low. I had to struggle to work every day to take care of my patients, deliver babies, and perform surgeries. In addition to these duties, I had to take care of my daughter, who was three years old.

Mentally I was anxious, depressed, and tired. Financially, I had to struggle. Spiritually, it was like falling in deep dark well; I felt like I could hardly breathe. That winter was awful; I did not know where my life was going.

Struggling to raise my daughter by myself and practice medicine, I had to send her to board at kindergarten full time. I took her on my bike to kindergarten at 6 AM every Monday and took her back at 6 PM on Saturday (we worked six days a week at that time). She was on my bike anywhere I went, no matter it was raining or snowing, 100F degrees, or 30F degrees. She got used to the "bike ride," and somehow, she liked it. On the weekend, I took her to parks, to go shopping, and do whatever I could to let her see new things. She and I were perfect friends. Sometimes when I was too busy, I would take her to her grandparents' home and let her stay there for several days. Whatever she liked, I would buy for her no matter how expensive; I wanted to make up for two parents love and care. I tightened my spending because I only had less than 100 Yuan per month ($15.00), and part of my income pay had to for her full-time kindergarten. When my husband passed, he left nothing; no bank account, no cash even though everyone knew he had a lot of money. I was not a "money girl" and never asked where his money was, or how much he had. I married him because I loved him. His sister-in-law (brother's wife) borrowed 2000 Yuan from him to have facial surgery, which was to make eyelid double so that she would look prettier. Since I did not have enough money to raise my daughter, I asked her to return some money to me. But she refused to give it back. I realized I had to do everything by myself. Fortunately, I had a lot of friends and family who helped me if I needed help. Their help and support certainly made a difference in my life. Some friends made clothes for my daughter. Sometimes my sisters took care of her; some friends took her overnight if I had a night shift to work in the hospital. Some of them took care of her weekends if I had to work. Some invited us for dinner, so I did not have to spend money and time on food. They did this all with love, care, kindness, and compassion. I was so grateful for having good friends and my family members who helped me in my difficult time, but still, I was very sad and lonely in my heart after losing him. I wished that the rest of my life would be more comfortable. I wanted someone in my life who would turn everything around and take care of me for the rest of my life.

A wish is a wish, and not every dream can come true, that I understood. Those days were my most challenging time, financially, physically, emotionally, but I did not ask for any money from anyone. I wanted to deal with life myself. I wanted to see how strong I could be. One month later, the Chinese New Year arrived. That was also a difficult time for me.

In China, Chinese New Year is the most important holiday of the year. People celebrate this holiday for 7 to 10 days, depending on your employer. Some companies gave more vacation days than others. On this big holiday, the family gets together and makes big meals every day. Every family cooks the best and most special dishes and other good food to celebrate the biggest event of the year. It is even more significant than Christmas and Thanksgiving because everyone in China celebrates this holiday (not everyone celebrates Christmas or Thanksgiving in America). In the Chinese tradition, the family gets together on Chinese New Year's Eve to make dumplings. During this time, everyone will be working together, joking, laughing, talking, teasing, and eating a lot of snacks. It's the best time. Making dumplings also involves "teamwork."

In our family, many years ago, we would have a "concert" every year. I played the Yang Qin, (a Chinese hammered dulcimer), my younger brother played the flute or the accordion, my sister played "Erhu" (a Chinese two-string instrument), my other sister sang, as did my older brother. My older brother was like a comedian, and he knew how to make people laugh. When the clock struck midnight, our family would light fireworks. Other families who had no fireworks would just come out to watch the fireworks and enjoy the fun together. After the fireworks, everyone went back home and started to cook the dumplings. Some families would cook different foods, and eat dumplings as a first New Year's meal. On New Year's Day (day one), the family would have a big dinner together, so this was a "cooking day." On day two and day three, there were "inter-family visiting days." Relatives would go to visit each other. If my sister's family visited me, my family members and I would be a "cooking team" and cook the best food for the visitors. On days four and five, there was "friends visiting day." You would go to visit anyone close to you, including the people who work for you or with you. On days six and seven, you start clean up or relax a little, get ready to go back to work. So Chinese New Year is a holiday that everyone would look forward to at the end of the year. But it was not fun for me this year.

I requested to work every day on this Chinese New Year holiday. But the director in the OB department wanted me to take it easy on this holiday. She did not give me a full schedule working on the holiday; she thought she was doing the right thing and doing me a favor. That made it difficult because I did not want to see anyone on this holiday. I thought some "busy work" might keep me distracted from being lonely and sad about losing my husband. My sisters and brothers all invited me to their houses for the holiday. I turned them down. I knew I would feel sad and cry if I went there and saw them. I felt like I didn't have a complete family.

One of my friends knew another friend, who was a bus driver (a small bus). He asked me if I would like to help him over the holiday selling tickets on the bus. I accepted his offer because I had no place to go on this holiday. I didn't want to stay home either. I sent my daughter to her grandparent's house then started five days of working on the bus selling tickets. On the bus, I wore sunglasses and a surgical mask to disguise myself. I didn't want people to recognize me. I was a doctor and had many patients nearby. Fortunately, no one did recognize me.

I worked from 8 AM to 11 PM for five days. I made 100 Yuan ($12.50). That wasn't a lot of money, but it certainly took my loneliness away. I wasn't just working for money anyway. Selling tickets all day long, I did not have time to think about anything. But at night, when I went back home, my mind would still trouble me. I carried the grief for many months.

I made 100 Yuan in 5 days. That could be somebody's monthly salary. I realized that I had to keep myself busy all of the time to avoid feeling sad and lonely. I decided to use the 100 Yuan for tuition to go to night school to study English. At that time, I had no reason for studying English; it was just something to keep myself busy. I knew that I always enjoyed my language study. I was pretty good with it in school. I was the assistant teacher when I was studying Russian language in junior high and high school.

The decision to go to night school to study English had significant consequences. It was soon to change the course of my life completely.

Chapter 10: Keep Learning and Life Changes

I signed up for evening English classes with a Science Institute in Changsha. The institute had foreign teachers; most of the teachers were from America. I did this for several reasons. First, I liked language study; I did very well with my composition class in high school and received A's often. Sometimes the teacher would read my composed article to the whole class. English is a different language, but since I liked all my language studies, it did not matter which language anymore. Second, I needed some distraction from the sadness, grief, and loneliness that I was experiencing. Lastly, I always like to learn. It doesn't matter what I learn, as long as it is useful and can enrich my life. Learning is a significant component of my life. I often choose to learn over playing cards (Chinese love to play cards, and it is a part of socializing too).

There were over 30 people in my class. Most students were engineers, teachers, technicians, doctors, or someone who had a prospect to go abroad. No matter what reason, these people wanted to be able to have conversations with foreigners to use their English.

There were four of us who got along very well; we were somehow attracted to each other. Therefore, we often discussed how we could learn English an efficient way. Among the four of us, there were two guys (one engineer, one scientist), one girl (teacher), and me (a practicing physician). The four of us were dedicated students and studied very hard, and soon we were able to have some conversations with each other in English. I thought we were the most intelligent and hard-working people in the class. We discussed many times going to a hotel where there were foreigners to practice speaking "real English" so that we would be able to speak correctly. One evening, we finally made this happen.

We all met at the Lotus Hotel in Changsha. At that time, the Lotus Hotel was the best hotel in Changsha City we thought it must have English speakers. The four of us met at 8 PM in the lobby of the hotel. Several foreigners were sitting in the cafe, but we didn't know who spoke English. In China, foreigners come from many different countries, including many Europeans. To us, they all looked alike. Since I had my daughter with me, I asked the others (classmates) to speak to the foreigners first. They were very shy and afraid to speak first. I realized that we were wasting time, and we all had to work the next day; therefore, I decided to break the "ice." I went up to an older woman and gently asked her, "Excuse me, do you speak English?" She was pleased to see someone talking to her and delighted to speak to me, "Yes, I do! How do you do". In China, at the time, people didn't talk to strangers. She was thrilled that I spoke to her. I sensed that she was lonely by herself in this very different country.

She then told me she was American and came to China for sightseeing. She was in her 80's, but she looked as if she was seventy-something. I explained that we were an English study group and came to the hotel to practice English with "real English-speaking people." I was glad to know that she could help us. My English classmates saw that I started the conversation with her; they came over right away, and sat down, occupying the rest of the three remaining seats. They were so happy and started a conversation with her immediately. There were only four seats around the table; there was no chair left for my daughter and me. Since I did not have a place, I told my classmate that I would find another table to sit. Since I had started the first conversation, my fear of speaking was smaller. I saw another foreigner sitting at a different table with coke in front of him, and I went over to ask him the same thing "Excuse me, do you speak English." I told him exactly the same thing as I had explained to the older lady. I told him who we were and why we were in the hotel. He was pleased that I spoke to him and asked me to have a seat. My daughter and I then sat down.

Before we started our polite conversation, my daughter told me that she wanted a coke. The coke cost 4 yuan (yuan is the Chinee dollar), but I only made 75 Yuan a month, even with the monthly bonus I still made less than 100 Yuan. I hesitated and wanted to explain to her to buy a can of coke in hotel cost too much money, and I could get it for her some other time for less money. But she was only three years old, and absolutely would not understand this situation. I did not want to show my status to this foreign stranger, nor did I want to waste time. Therefore, I bought her the coke, trying to be a good mother even though I felt it was not worth it to pay 4 Yuan to buy a can of coke. She was delighted to drink her coke; I was happy to focus on my learning.

My English was not good at all, but we had a pleasant conversation, mostly due to his patience. He told me that he was from America and had come to Chang Sha to train some people at a local computer factory. At that time, computers were starting to become popular. He was very patient and spoke to me slowly so that I could understand easily. Sometimes he referred a small dictionary that he had with him to help our conversation. Since he had been on many trips to China, he was used to hearing "Chinese English." We had a good conversation even though my language was limited. I realized many questions I asked him at that time were not exactly proper to ask due to our cultural difference. But I did not know until later, after living in the US and learning the culture.

Before we said good-bye, he asked me if we could meet again. I hesitated but agreed to meet him in a public park nearby the Lotus Hotel. I did not want to meet a stranger in a private place, so I gave him directions to Xiao Yuan Park. We met at Xiao Yuan Park the next day after work and had a lovely time and conversation. I was brave enough to ask many more questions from the "English 900" (900 questions and answers in English), and he was kind enough to answer all the questions I asked. We seemed to have no problem talking to each other (we both carried a pocket dictionary). Before we said goodbye, he asked me if he could see my apartment. He said that in all his travels to China, he was always staying in hotels and was not able to see what "Chinese homes" were like. I hesitated because I had one room in an apartment building in the hospital where I was working, no kitchen, no bathroom, everything in one small room. It was not typical. I also had my daughter with me.

Additionally, my sister and her son were in my apartment at the time because her son had broken his leg and was being treated at my hospital. They were staying in my place most of the time, and my apartment was tiny. On the other hand, it would be safe because my sister and her son were there. So, I agreed to have him come to my apartment the next day.

His name is Gerry. He came to my apartment the next day. That evening, he found out that my husband had passed away, from a picture hanging on the wall. He showed great sympathy and compassion. We had a pleasant evening conversation and talked about many more things. He seemed sincere and kind, a nice person to be a friend. He did not tell me that my apartment was too small, neither care about no bathroom, no other things. After he left, my sister expressed he was a nice person, polite, good manners, and a gentleman. I agreed, but who knew what the truth was, it always takes time to know a person well.

Before leaving, he asked if he could write to me when he got back to the US. At that time, I did not believe him, because we had just met, and he was just an acquaintance. Anybody would say the same thing to be polite and friendly. I said yes but did not have any expectations. After one month, I was surprised to receive his letter from the USA; he did write a letter to me after all!

We became pen pals for a while, and we kept our distant friendship. One letter I received from him was exciting; he said he would come back to do more work in China and would like to visit me again. Somehow, I was delighted and excited hearing this news, feeling like a good friend kept his word. Six months later, we met again in Changsha. We were happy to see each other. On this visit, we talked much more and started to get to know each other more and more, better and better. My English was a little better too. I felt he was a kind, sincere, honest, good-hearted, caring, and loving person. We started to have more casual conversations, teasing each other, but still in a friendly manner. I took him to Martyr Park in Changsha. Martyr Park is the largest park in Changsha, and many people enjoy hanging out there for a stroll, jogging, exercise, singing, play games, play instruments, photo shooting, eating, boating, painting, dancing, and many other activities.

We walked along the lake in Martyr Park, looking at the beautiful lake, trees, birds, boats, and noticing that people were staring at us. At that time, not many foreigners visited Changsha, and every foreigner got a lot of attention from the locals. It was a little intimidating at the time. I was relieved to think that those staring at me probably just thought I was his interpreter, luckily.

I also took him to the bank of the Xiang Jiang river, which is branch Yang Zi river. We visited a lot of my friends and some other places in Changsha. We had a great time. On this trip, a stronger relationship began to develop.

Gerry and I became good friends. He came to China 10 times between 1986 and 1987 and learned a lot about Chinese culture and a little bit of the Chinese language. He told me that many things about the Chinese culture were interesting to him, including many things that surprised him too. The two countries were so different, which was the reason he was excited and had a new feeling. We were often laughing and joking, especially about cultural differences. On this trip, he stayed in China for nine days, so we were able to spend some good times together in public places. We developed feelings for each other and knew something was happening between us. I started to test my family to see their response to our strange relationship. It was immediately rejected. My family asked me not to trust a foreigner. Especially my father, a Communist Party member for a long time, always thinking America is an "Imperialist Country," "an enemy to China." My family was so afraid that I would be tricked or played.

I started to talk to my friends about this. They were also surprised to know I was so close to this person in such a short time. They began to ask questions: "How do you know if he is single?"

"What if he has AIDS?" "How do you know he is an honest person?" "How do you know he is a nice person"? "What makes you trust him"? "What about if he gets tired of you and leaves"? "How do you know if he has enough money to support you"? "What would happen if he has no money and you don't speak English, you cannot work"? "What if he has a wife in America"? "How do you know he will take care of you"? There were millions of questions from my family and my friends. I knew in my heart that they just wanted me to be safe and happy.

All my family and my friends were beginning to worry about me. None of them stayed on my side. It was hard to choose between my family, my friends, and him. Who should I believe? My sixth sense told me that he was the right person, and very often, my sixth-sense got me to the best place in the past. One day I decided to do a little test on him. It did not seem to strike him as important, but it meant a lot to me, and it certainly helped me make my decision. I asked him: "If there were three girls you could date, the first one very pretty with a beautiful body, the second one very intelligent, and the third one has nothing but honesty, which one would you chose"? He answered my question: "the girl who is honest but has no money." It struck me right away; he earned my trust. (You can see how innocent I was). I was thinking, if he prefers honesty, he may be an honest person.

I felt he was the right person (even though it was somewhat naïve of me to think this way). I started to consider the situation very deeply and carefully. I analyzed where I was at the time: I did have a good job, good friends, and family, but I did not like China's corrupted government. I did appreciate my family and my friend's concern and care for me, I did see the points they made, but I liked him, I wanted to be with him, and I felt safe with him. I felt so in love and felt a tie between him and I. My feelings were powerful at that time. I then started to reason with myself. First of all, I am the one who should make choices in my life. Second, I could not live with my family forever; I should live with the person I love. Then I started to answer the questions my friends and my family had: "What if something happened between us?....... I would find a job to support my child and myself". "If he was not the person I loved and could live with, or not the right person for me, I would find my way out"; "What if he tricks you or abandons you? I would go to the Chinese embassy for help" .... I was able to answer every question my family and my friends had placed in my head.

I could not sleep for many nights. I wanted to be sure that I made the right choice because I had to give up everything I had in China (at that time I was 31 years old) and had all I needed: my work, my friends, my parents, my siblings. My father was upset and asked me, "There are millions of Chinese men, why do you have to love and marry a foreigner"? I did not want to answer the question because I was in love.

I made up my mind to go forward with Gerry. I made up my mind that I was going to discover a new life, to have a middle-age adventure. I have always believed that if you put in enough effort, anything can change even a stone can change its shape. I also felt that life should be better and better, not worse and worse. My instinct told me this is the nature of life, and I will be fine.

On September 26, 1988, we got our marriage certificate from the City. On October 1, we got married in China and had a Chinese wedding. That was a real adventure for us. My parents did not come to the wedding (they were angry with me), and so I asked my aunt and uncle to come to be the "parents" at my wedding. I couldn't say much about it, but I thought that my parents were a little unfair to me, but I knew they had their reasons, and I believe they loved me and cared for me no matter what. About 70 people attended our wedding (mainly my friends and family), and everyone had a good time. Everyone seemed to like him. My aunt and my uncle did an excellent job being my "parents." Everything had gone well.

Four months after the wedding, I got my visa. Gerry came to China again and brought my daughter and me to the United States. On February 17, 1989, we landed in the United States. I described it as my "unfamiliar country," my "new dream country." Now, my new adventure and my new life began.

Part II: A Challenging Journey in the USA

Chapter 11: Living in the States

Before I came to the US, I was still working in the hospital. When my belly was getting bigger, it was apparent to see I was pregnant. The hospital official told me I needed to have an abortion if I wanted to keep my job. I was distraught; I wanted to keep my baby but also wanted to keep the job. But I could not say anything because in China at that time there was a national policy, "One child per family." I did not know how long it would take for me to get a visa, but I had to tell the hospital leaders that I planned to leave China soon. They asked me when I would be going, what date and month. I believe if I didn't have the answer, they might fire me from the hospital right away. I told the hospital that the visa was in process, and I will leave as soon as I got the permission. In the meantime, my new husband was working very hard to get the visa work done for us to come to the US. I wrote to him and called him to say, "Hurry Up!" I did not explain why he needed to hurry to get the visa. With the pressure from the hospital, I wanted to get out of there. Every time I saw them, the first question was, "When do you leave?" Finally, I decided to quit the job before I got the visa because they were asking me the same question too often, and I could not deal with it anymore. I was upset. In China in those days, many things were upsetting, and people had to deal with it. They felt it was a part of life. But I did not want to deal with it anymore, and I wanted to keep my dignity, so I quit. As soon as I quit my job, I felt much more relaxed. Several months later, I came to America, the beautiful land.

I first lived in Maryland when I came to the United States, just 30 minutes from Washington, DC. Gerry was working for a company doing business with China, and his job was to train Chinese technicians on how to use computer-related equipment. I was six months pregnant with our son Peter.

Living in America was much more comfortable than living in China. We had a three-floor townhouse in Maryland with a big master bedroom, two and a half bathrooms, and a big living room. There was no comparison to living in China at that time. In China at that time, housing was owned by the government, and any worker's apartment was arranged by the company, factory, institute, school, wherever you were working. In the US, anyone can buy a home if you have enough for a down payment. The living situation was much better in the US.

Even though I was comfortable living in a real condo home, in the beginning, I could not get used to all of the differences in this new country. I felt lonely, bored, didn't see people either on the street or anywhere in this rural neighborhood. I had no social interaction. Part of the reason was that I was pregnant six months when I got here. I could not do much, could not go to many places, did not speaking English well, and couldn't drive yet. The cultural difference and the language barrier were still significant obstacles for many things. People seemed cold; neighbors didn't talk to each other, not like in China, where the people were friendly, especially neighbors and friends. Nothing was convenient in the place I lived; you could not go anywhere on foot. Not much was within walking distance. In China, many places I could easily walk to or bike there, and many department stores and grocery stores and markets were within walking distance. It was very convenient. My new place was not centrally-located. I was somewhat isolated, and I lacked the interaction with other people that I was so used to in China.

I was determined to get used to my "new world." There is an old saying in Chinese "Ru Xiang Sui Shu," which means "If you just arrived and planned to live in a new village, you go with the custom/routine of this village." I kept telling myself, "it will be better, and I will get used to the different life." I focused on taking care of my daughter Sharon and teaching my daughter English. We started to watch "Sesame Street" together so that we could both learn English at the same time. Sesame Street was a TV show for young children. My daughter learned much faster than I did. But I wanted to keep learning the language. I wanted to be able to ask questions so that I could get to know this new culture and hopefully get used to this new life. I tried to read the newspaper, but it was not easy with all the new words, and complicated sentence structure, and all those little definite articles and prepositions, etc. I wanted to go to school to study English, but there was no way I could do that. I had two young children (my son was born three months later), didn't speak much English, and had to take care of my husband and the house. I was not a superwoman. So, I had to let go of going to school, but I could still learn English by myself while taking care of everything. Therefore, I did it, but not that well.

In the first month living in DC, my husband took me to a Chinese restaurant called "Hunan Restaurant." He thought I came from Hunan, should be very happy to know there was a Hunan restaurant in the city. We had our first "Hunan Meal" in DC. It was not Hunan food, not even close to Hunan food. I was disappointed, but there was nothing I could do except to cook myself and make real Chinese food for all of us. Before, I was the worst chef in my family, and all my sisters and brothers are much better than me. Within several months, my cooking skills became much better, and my husband did not want to go to Chinese restaurants anymore. I guess anyone can do anything if they are determined.

Sometimes we went to a western-style restaurant. I was shocked to see people eating a colossal piece steak, which I could cut up, do stir fry and mix with some vegetables to feed the whole family. I realized the considerable cultural differences to which I would need to adapt. I may not necessarily need to follow their diet, but I should not criticize it.

After just one month of living in the new place, my husband had to leave for an overseas business trip for a week. That was very difficult. He was the only person I knew. He didn't want me to feel lonely, so he brought my daughter and me to his relative's house in another state to stay for a week. He has a sweet family, but since our culture was so different, there were some misunderstandings between his relatives and I. In China, the host always offers the best meal and other food to the guests, even if the host has very little (financially) to offer. They like to take care of the guest by making the guest comfortable; they don't mind working hard. They want to show their hospitality. My first lunch in his relative's house was a hot dog. I was surprised. I felt insulted and mistreated. I thought perhaps they didn't like my daughter and me. In another relative's house, I was served "Ramen Noodles" for lunch. I thought that was a joke. In China, people would eat "Ramen Noodle" when they have no food to eat in the house or no time to cook. That is also the cheapest meal. In China, food is a big thing, and everyone likes to eat good tasting food. I then really missed my family and my friends; I was never treated that way before. I thought Americans are so cheap, they made much more money than Chinese, but unwilling to spend on food for their guests.

When my husband came back from his business trip, I expressed my feelings. I told him that I wasn't happy, I felt mistreated, I felt insulted, I felt the prejudice. He was very patient with me and told me there is a significant cultural difference between China and the United States. He told me that if people don't give you a delicious meal, it doesn't mean they don't like you. Some people don't want to spend time to cook, or don't have time to prepare a meal, or don't know what the guest might like. Some people always eat this way and don't treat others differently. Most of all, they have no concept of what food you ate in China. From his explanation, I then realized that I had to accept the cultural difference. I knew it would take time to get used to it, but I was determined to make changes in my way of thinking, remove my negative thoughts, and to go with it.

About one month before I gave birth to my son, we visited Gerry's family again. It was the first time I experienced a surprise baby shower. It was a very warm, friendly, happy, and joyful atmosphere, I got so many gifts to use for the baby, and I had a great time. This kindness and the surprise party touched me. That changed my thoughts from negative to positive. I, once again, realized that I had so much to learn and so much that I needed to improve.

Three months after coming to the US, I gave birth to my son Peter. That was a scary experience. I did not know the doctor well enough to trust. I felt like they were going to kill me or injure me. I screamed and was very anxious during the delivery process; they had to use IV anesthesia to knock me out. When I heard my son's first cry, I finally burst into tears, not sure if they were tears of joy or tears of relief. I could not believe I was safe, and I was alive. It turned out everything was excellent, and it was only me who carried so much anxiety, fear, not knowing the culture, and having no family support. Compared to Chinese hospitals where there were no private rooms for regular people, this hospital in Washington DC was in much better condition and had much better services. I had a private room and bath, and it was all positive in the end. There was no reason for me to panic. It just wasted my energy and surely showed how anxious I was those days.

I had to stay home to take care of my son and my daughter. In China, a woman could take 2 to 4 months off from work to stay home after giving birth. During these months, there are often visits from family and friends, and that makes time go by fast; the social time with visitors takes away the loneliness for the mother. Living in Maryland, I was very lonely and troubled. In China, I had always been busy working with practicing medicine in the hospital, never did I have such a quiet time. I did not know anyone besides my daughter, my husband, and my newborn son. I could not drive, could not go out without my husband. I missed my family very much.

In China, I never heard of "postpartum depression." Living in this country for a while, especially after I had my holistic medicine clinic, I treated many patients who suffered with "postpartum depression," When I think back, I think I may have had postpartum depression.

I needed to help myself to get past these feelings, so I decided to spend more time with the self-study of English by trying to memorize more vocabulary. Also, watching PBS programs on TV with my daughter, I spent time reading whatever books I could find while the children were sleeping. I noticed both of us (my daughter and I) experienced homesickness and mild depression. I struggled against it by trying to read more, trying to go out to meet people, trying to get some information about everything. One bit of information I got from a neighbor was how to get a license to practice medicine in this country. That was positive. I realized there was hope for me.

After living in Maryland for six months, my husband got a new job in Massachusetts. I had my first moving experience. I never had so much stuff in China, and I had to learn packing/unpacking, putting things away. I was not good at doing this. After this moving experience, I told myself and my husband, "I never want to move again!"

Moving to MA did not make things better. We now had a house and a yard; therefore, I was busy with housework, learning English, and taking care of the children. But my postpartum depression was improved because I was "busy." I didn't realize how difficult things would be without strong English language skills. It was hard to do anything. I was still feeling insecure, afraid to speak, felt useless, not much joy in life besides housework, but I did have pleasure from being with my children. I was determined to take good care of my children and make sure they grew healthy and happy.

To learn English and medical terminology, I decided to find a job in the local hospital. Fortunately, I found a part-time job as a medical secretary and assistant in the OB/GYN ward at the hospital. That was somewhat naive and a mistake. My job was to answer the phone and put patient's information and doctor's orders into the computer. The first challenge was answering the phone. People often spoke so fast that I could hardly understand. Many callers (either patients or family members of patients) used slang that I didn't understand at all. Many times I had to ask the nurses to help me, even though I hated to do that. Some nurses were kind and patient; others were very impatient, some even rude. I kept telling myself: I need to stay, I need to learn English, learn medical words, learn things in this hospital. I needed to deal with these difficulties; I needed to persevere and compromise. I hated this job, and I was not qualified to take this job because my language was so limited. By hiring me, the hospital was doing me a favor. My mind was not in the right place, and I was thinking negatively: I use to tell the nurses what to do when I was practicing medicine in China; now everyone was telling me what to do. I use to be an excellent OB-GYN, had a good relationship with patients, nurses, and other staff working with me, now I could hardly have a decent conversation with any of them. I used to have a good reputation with my skills; now, I knew nothing, could not do anything, not even the most straightforward job. I felt useless. I felt life was not fair; all my knowledge and clinical experience in medical care were wasted. I was depressed again, mainly from my cynical mind. I was too negative, and I did not have any guidance toward a positive way of living.

One day, a doctor asked me to put his prescription into the computer. I could not read this doctor's hand-writing. So, I asked him what the spelling was on this prescription. He made fun of me and made me feel bad about this job. I was very uncomfortable. I felt insulted. I tried to be patient, but it did not last long. I got help from a nurse to read this prescription. Right after I put the correct name of the drug into the computer, I left work and never returned. The next day when the nurse manager called me, I confirmed that I would not return to the hospital. My feelings were hurt so badly. Six-months working in that hospital was torture for me. Every minute was uncomfortable. I told myself if there is a chance, I could be a doctor again, I would never do this to anyone no matter what. I was unhappy and insecure; I didn't feel like I fit in anywhere. I did not have much wisdom, either. I was wrapped up in these emotional struggles. But at least I had my family: my husband, my daughter, and my son.

But now thinking it over, it was not anyone's fault; it was me who was not able to adapt to the situation and the differences. It was me who could not take criticism; it was me who was not patient in learning life's lessons and having such a quick temper that caused my making the wrong decision. I still had a lot to learn and a lot of growing to do.

Everything has two sides: the Yin side and the Yang side. When I look back at those experiences working in the hospital, I did learn something. I learned some medical terminology; I learned how American hospitals work, how American doctors deal with patients and nurses, how much work and pressure the nurses had to deal with, and how much paperwork every staff member had to handle. And how much waste there was in the hospital. I now realize it wasn't a bad experience but rather a learning experience. That is one of the many ways to learn about life: Go through a hard time before a good time.

I started to think seriously about my future in this strange and new country. I decided to go for the examination from the National Board of Medicine. If I passed the test, I could become a doctor and practice medicine in this country. I would have a decent income if I became a doctor, I would not be feeling bad about myself anymore, and I would not have to deal with negative feelings anymore. My dream might come true. But those thoughts, as I now think back, were only temporary comfort.

Shortly after I left the hospital, I found a job working at UMass Medical Center researching Aids. My boss was a very nice man and treated me well. I was happier doing research work: nobody bothers me, nobody criticizes me, and no prejudice because many on the research staff were from other countries. I was pleased just to be doing my work.

Shortly after I started working, my husband lost his job. We had just bought a house and had a big mortgage. My husband was very nervous and upset, which did not make my life easy. I was beginning to have a more comfortable life, and here I had to live with an angry man daily. I said to him: if we lose the house, we can move to an apartment; what is the big deal? He replied: I worked and saved so hard to buy a house; I don't want to lose it. Then I decide to work two jobs: full time working at UMass Medical school and part-time working in a Chinese restaurant. Which means, I worked 40 hours Monday through Friday, and Friday evening and Saturday and Sunday I worked in the restaurant. As you see, I had no break. But that was alright as long as I didn't have to deal with the negative emotions. At least my husband could take care of the children these days. At this challenging time, all my thoughts were about how to support our family. A year later, I quit the restaurant work when my husband again found a job.

After a while working in the medical lab, I started to have a headache. I felt the chemicals I was dealing with affected me and caused problems. I thought, tough it up and the headaches may go away. But my troubles continued. I may have had allergies to some of those chemicals. But at that time, I did not know for sure. Finally, I decided not to do research anymore. Many years later, I found out from a blood test that I do have a lot of allergies.

I made up my mind up to move forward and take the examination with the Board of Medicine. I bought all the necessary materials and started this hard journey. The language was a significant barrier, these were all courses that I had already studied in medical school, but now it was in a different language. Some courses were new to me, but most courses were familiar except that now there was new medical terminology I had to memorize. That was a very dull and intense study. I was exhausted every day.

At that time, my daughter was in 1st grade, and my son was two years old. I spent so much time studying and did not pay much attention to my children. One day, my daughter brought home a class picture to show me. Suddenly my tears poured down like a stream when I looked at this picture: All girls and boys were dressed nicely except my daughter, who was wearing a T-shirt and had messy hair. My heart sank and was broken at that moment, and I felt so guilty and embarrassed, so sad. I thought that I wasn't doing the mother's job. I wasn't a good mother even though I was trying my best to be one. I suddenly decided to quit my studies and let go of my plan to take the examination. I let go of my desire to become a doctor in this country. I could not handle seeing my children were not being cared for, looking like orphaned children. I needed to take better care of my children; they needed me. I didn't care about making big money. I didn't care about future fame. Now, I just wanted to be a good mother. So, I quit my study for the board exam.

I gave up my dream to become an American Doctor. I then felt so relieved and relaxed, and I could breathe. I spent more time with my family and my children, spent some time with new friends I met. I enjoyed garden work, arts, and crafts work, practiced my exercise, took my kids out to parks, museums, children's playgrounds, and visiting other people, just like a good mother.

I did not waste my time during those days of study. I learned a lot of medical terminologies; I refreshed my knowledge of medicine; I learned new things when I was studying because certain diseases were rare in China but common in the United States, and other diseases were common in China but rare in the US. Life is never self-evident, sometimes you feel you lost something, but in reality, you gained. You gain from loss; you learn from failure. You appreciate more after you go through a hard time. I certainly did. I later became a holistic doctor who not only helped many patients but also helped myself and my family.

My children are good kids, and both of them completed college and are on their journey with career and hobbies. No matter where they are, I always love them. My daughter is brilliant; quick-thinking had excellent grades in school and never made me worry about her homework. She was well organized, structured, always followed the rules, and has good work ethics. She was an excellent violin player and had one time played as the first violin in a school concert. She also had some leadership skills, which later helped her become a good teacher in both ballroom dancing and violin.

My son was adorable when he was a baby. He had lovely fat cheeks during his childhood that everyone wanted to pinch him to the point he hated it. He was friendly, has excellent people skills, a pleasant personality, and he is smart too. He is a musician but also very much into physical training nowadays.

During those times taking care of them and raising them, I felt challenges. Taking care of children is not hard; just doing what a mother is supposed to do: feed them well, take them to places, do activities. But raising children is different. As I did raise my kids and was taking care of the family, I learned so much. One of the most challenging things I found living in America was raising kids. In China, we all raise kids the same way; we all felt we knew how to raise our kids. We teach the kids about listening to parents, never arguing with parents, always helping parents anytime they need it. We teach them about doing what parents ask and taking care of their parents when they were not well or when they are getting older. But it seemed so hard raising kids in the US. It was so different, and I was puzzled and confused about my ability to raise my kids. I sometimes explained to them about the Chinese culture of how children should behave, how they should not talk back, how children obey parents. But they would argue with me, "Mom, this is America, not China." They were right, but I was not raised here and did not understand how to raise kids in the US.

In their school days, I did not realize that my kids experienced peer pressure and prejudice. (I did not know this until my son was 29 and told me). We did not have these issues in China. At the time, I had to struggle to make a living, which consumed much of my time. My kids were experiencing emotional issues that I did not even know about; I worked too hard and too much. I thought just giving them what they wanted should be fine. I was not thinking clearly. I did not stop them from watching TV at dinner time; I did not force my son to stop playing video games so much. I now wish I spent more time with them, to teach them, to be more patient with them, and to pay more attention to their emotional health.

During these years of taking care of my family and raising my children, I had a small business selling medical equipment to China from the USA. I sold one piece of equipment to a manufacturer in China, but I decided to quit soon after. I never trained in business, and I was not interested in selling or marketing. Re-assessing my strengths, I think my characteristics are: soft-hearted, kind, compassionate, eager to help people get well, and caring about people. So, I decided to change my direction.

While searching for my path, I had many thoughts looking at the whole picture of living in the States. The bottom line was that I wanted to use my skills to help people. "How" I could help people, would be the starting point of my journey. Since I had lived in two different countries, experienced two separate lives, I realized that the medical care system in the United States was not complete; something was missing. In China, there are two types of medicine that people can choose: conventional medicine and traditional Chinese medicine. Most people know how to choose their medical care; they know when to use conventional medicine and when to use Chinese medicine. It works very well. But here in the US, it seemed there was no choice. I wished there was more quality care from doctors. I always liked to do things naturally, and don't want to take medication unless it is necessary. I believe that we come from nature; nature has the power to give us sickness and also make us well.

In medical school, we studied both Conventional (western) Medicine and Traditional Chinese medicine. I experienced using both treatments myself, and I practiced using both on my patients when I was in China. I know precisely what both modalities can do for your body and how they work. But living here in the US, I had very little chance to get help naturally at that time. If I went to a doctor, almost every doctor prescribes medications to target the symptoms. I understood that was how they trained, and prescribing medication is very common. I even did it myself when I was working in the hospital and clinic. Unfortunately, sometimes, the medicines didn't work. At that time (in the US), many doctors didn't try to look for choices for patients. They didn't look into what was going on in the physical body, along with emotional health. They did they look for what was the cause of the problem or the root of the problem. Some of them had a narrow mind and vision. There is a Chinese expression, "the frog sitting in the well looking at the sky" (how much sky can you see?). They spent so little time with each patient and then gave medications and sent them home. Some of them listen to you for two minutes then decide what you have. When you have pain or illness, they rarely ask you anything else besides where the pain is, how severe the pain is; then, a prescription is provided to patients. Without finding causes, just using a pain killer can only cover up the problem, not solve the problem. I feel many doctors don't have plans for patients to improve their health. They don't talk about how to prevent illnesses. They completely ignore the two most essential parts of human healing, the "human energy" and the "mind-body connection."

The human body is a big mystery and is much more complicated than we know. I have been a doctor since 1982, but I still feel I have a lot to learn about the human body, connection between mind and body, and healing. I started to read more books about holistic healing and mind-body medicine. I went back to China many times to talk to many different doctors who were experts in traditional Chinese medicine and Masters of Qi Gong, Tai Chi. It opened my mind, and my heart and I accumulated more knowledge of natural healing. Disease and healing involve many things, such as lifestyle, exercise, diet and eating habits, living environment, emotional state, workload, stress level, daily activities, mindset, personality, sexual activity, personal hygiene, etc. But doctors in conventional medicine have minimal time to discuss these; therefore, they don't know how to heal, but they do know how to save lives and provide symptomatic relief.

I still remembered in early 1978, when the medical students came to school in the beginning, our Principle gave us a speech, he said: "We are here to learn how to save lives, heal the injured or sick. The quality of care for our patients is our first purpose (goal). You do the best you can to help the patients, healing with your heart". The day I entered medical school, I decided to help people to the best of my ability.

Now, I suddenly felt a sense of joy because I made my decision to become a holistic doctor who could help people to heal, to feel better truly, to restore their health and happiness. I wanted to be the real deal; I wanted to help people who desperately needed to find a cure, and I wanted to be the one who had the particular skills they needed. I decided to go back to China to continue my studies in holistic medicine.

Looking back at my life in the US, there were so many good things: clean country, fresh air, beautiful environment, well-regulated and structured system, and most of all: the freedom of life, career, work, and living. But I did not focus on these, and I was too negative; I had a lot to learn, and I did learn.

Chapter 12: Journey to Holistic Medicine

I thought over and over about the systems in these two different countries: China had less comfortable living conditions, less income (at that time), fewer material possessions, but had more family bonds, more social life, more healthy food, more physical movement in daily life such as walking and biking to work. China had more support from family and friends. US had a better living situation, more income, but a more isolated culture; less help from friends and family, less social interaction, less walking more using the car when needing to go places. There is a big problem with drug issues and no right solution. With such a sedentary lifestyle, in addition to all the stress, people are not as healthy as they could be.

I wondered: What is my passion? What is my gift, what is the most substantial part of me? What are my weaknesses?

I am not good at fighting or auguring; don't like to compete with anyone. I cannot handle too much physical work, don't want to take any job just for making a living, not good with mechanical work, not good with too much paperwork (language barrier). I don't like to deal with people who are not honest or are rude, not very good at taking criticism (I am much better now). I'm not good at following orders doing things that are not ethical or not right. But I am a hard-working person, compassionate, sincere, open-minded, like to learn, like to improve, always want to make things better. I love life, enjoy being with people, like to help people to feel better, enjoy quiet time as well as fun time, and have a methodical mind.

I wanted to make a difference, to promote something healthier that might change things; I wanted to help people to improve their life and health because I know how important it is to feel good. How could I do this? I decided to teach, starting with exercises such as Tai Chi, Qi Gong. In medical school, we had Tai Chi classes, and I liked it. I also liked the Tai Chi Sword in the class. On my own, I studied Qi Gong but did not deeply understand it yet at that time. I only knew some people had great healing results. But being curious, I wanted to explore more, I wanted to have a deeper understanding of the power of Qi Gong, and why and how it is so effective.

I have always loved Chinese martial art. I studied sword exercise (martial art form) when I was ten years old, and some other martial arts in later years. In medical school, we also learned Tai Chi and Tai Chi sword. During the school year, I studied Qi Gong outside of school. I loved it because it made me feel so good. During my time practicing medicine in China, I organized and taught very successful wellness classes. I lost 20 lbs. teaching this particular exercise class, and other students enjoyed it too. Not only that, by teaching wellness classes in China, I gained teaching experience.

In 1992 living in Massachusetts, I started to teach in local facilities as well as having my classes. I just wanted to see what the results were. Amazingly, my students gave me fantastic feedback stating that their energy improved, emotion improved, physical pain reduced, blood pressure lowered, digestive function improved, anger reduced, balance improved, and they felt much happier. That was very encouraging because I was doing a study on my own and achieved such good results. Along with the healing effects, students were very appreciative of my teaching; they gave me pie, gifts, gave me so many hugs, and invited me to their homes.

I started to teach about a balanced diet, the mind-body connection, and the holistic approach in prevention and healing. Students asked me if I could see patients. At that time, I did not have my own office, but I wanted to continue to help people. I felt I needed to broaden my knowledge in traditional Chinese medicine and other natural therapies with a holistic approach; I wanted to be the best holistic doctor, one who can help patients to truly heal when they found no relief from other therapies or treatment.

I decided to go back to China to do more study and get more training. In early December 1995, I was accepted to work in a teaching hospital of Chinese medicine, which had the best reputation for TCM orthopedic medicine. I worked directly under the head doctor of each department, rotating in the different departments: acupuncture department, Tui Na/An Mo department, dermatology department, orthopedic department. I worked long hours even on holidays when other doctors wanted to have holidays off. I tried to get along with all the doctors, and hopefully, they would be willing to share their TCM (Traditional Chinese Medicine) knowledge with me. I invited all the doctors from all these departments for dinner to thank them for helping me to learn. It seems I was bribing them but with the good intention of learning. It worked! They treated me very well and helped me with herbal medicine, therapeutic techniques, tips, strategies, and how to deal with severe patient cases. I am thankful that I had this opportunity to learn, and I gained so much knowledge from this experience.

In China, while I was studying TCM, I was also studying Chen Style Tai Chi and Qi Gong with different masters. I worked from 8 am to 6 pm in the hospital, then study Tai Chi/Qi Gong afterward, every day except the weekend when I wanted to stay with my family. I worked too hard; I forced myself to do so because I wanted to make the most of my time in China. I lost the balance of my health, and I got very sick. I had bronchitis that turned into pneumonia. It was so bad I had to drag myself up every morning to go to work, I did not want to waste my time, so I continued to work except for one day when I had a fever and could not get up. At that time, I began hearing my own words again and again, "I would be pleased if I could get back to the US alive." The sickness lasted almost three weeks that hurt my energy. I was tired for another few weeks after that but still wanted to continue to work. I had not fully recovered before I went back to the US. I always appreciated the time I was there learning and practicing. I felt if I wanted to get something, I must have some losses. There is no such thing as "always winning."

I had my six-year-old son Peter with me on this trip. He went to grade school, where my sister was teaching. During the time I was in

China working in TCM hospital, my two sisters were taking care of him alternately. I am forever grateful to my sisters and other of my family members; I thank them forever for everything they did for me. I felt so lucky to have such a loving, caring, and giving family. Without their help, I could not have completed my journey in TCM study.

I had never studied business, but I started my own business in 1996, sharing an office with two other Doctors while living in Massachusetts. In 1997, I finally had my own private TCM clinic, "Chinese Medicine for Health," and the "New England School of Tai Chi." Lacking knowledge of how to do business, I had to take some classes, some training courses in marketing, business, accounting, managing, etc. I learned how to manage my business in addition to seeing patients, teaching classes, paying bills, hiring people, and letting go of people (that was the hardest part), etc. Of all of these, managing people is the most challenging thing, but over the years, I got better at it. Each day I would see 8 to 12 patients, then teach two classes in the evening. During the 17-years having the holistic healing business in Massachusetts, I taught many classes: Tai Chi, Tai Chi Sword, Tai Chi Fan, Tai Chi Stuff, various Qi Gong forms, Ba Gua, Xing Yi, Pushing Hands, and more. I worked 11 to 12 hours a day (too much). But my goal at that time was: I have to succeed! I cannot fail!

In 1999, with the help of a registered nurse who was also working for me at that time, I started to offer CEU (Continue Education Unit) programs for nurses. I am very much grateful for her help. In the United States, every several years, the nurses would need CE credits to continue their license. Two years later, I expended my CE program to physical therapists and occupational therapists. People enjoyed my CE programs very much, especially with my teaching model: Theory and practice. They enjoyed Qi Gong in the CE program. One nurse humorously told me, "Dr. Kuhn, this is the only program I did not fall to sleep"! She wanted to tell me how much she had enjoyed my program. It was a very successful CE program for six years. Later, I offered CE programs to massage therapists.

In 2004 I started offering training programs, such as a Tai Chi Instructor Training course and a Qi Gong Instructor Training Course. There were three reasons that I decided to start offering this training:

1. During the CE programs for nurses, some of the nurses felt so good after the program that they wanted to learn Qi Gong or Tai Chi so that they could teach their patients. These nurses sincerely wished to help their patients.

2. I had people tell me they had done Tai Chi before for x amount of years, but not until they came to my Tai Chi classes, did they get the Tai Chi principles. It was apparent to me: there was a need for well-trained Tai Chi teachers.

3. When I do patients consultation/treatment, I always teach some Qi Gong exercises targeted to the patient's illness. Since the results were so good, some therapists who were also working in wellness centers, or other holistic medicine clinics, wanted to learn Qi Gong not only to continue their healing but also to help their clients.

Later, when I was not able to find a good healing type massage therapy for my healing (I had many physical problems), I offered a wellness Tui Na therapy training course (also a CE course, for four years). In China, in the past, Tui Na therapy (a Chinese massage type) was offered only in hospitals for treating illness, but now is being provided in many clinics and wellness centers. This kind of hands-on therapy is very powerful, effective, comfortable, and most people in China love it. I not only studied Tui Na therapy in TCM hospital during the time I was there but also learned from different teachers in China. Every teacher had unique skills; I only use some of the techniques so that there is almost have no chance to injure anyone. Many people think the best healing is "No pain, no gain," but my approach is "No pain, but yes gain." So, I started to put together the most effective and safe Tui Na techniques, and these later became my Tui Na training course.

In my nationwide training programs, I have many students from different states and cities, some even from other countries. They are intelligent, kind, modest, hardworking, giving, passionate about learning and helping others, and have so many other good qualities. Working with my students, I always feel good and experience so much positive energy.

Practicing holistic medicine: I had so many different kinds of patients: teachers, doctors, lawyers, engineers, sales, computer worker, housewife, children, athletes, singers, actress, military people, nurses, PT, OT, banker, all different ethnic backgrounds such as black, white, Hispanic, middle eastern, central American, south American, European.... I have also seen many different characters such as greedy, selfish, egocentric, snobbish, also seeing many with kindness, gentleness, giving, loving, talented, happy, upbeat, loyal, friendly. Dealing with and having experience with all kinds of people, I learned a lot: learned to respect different cultures, to respond to various comments and criticisms, different ethnic diets, and the relation between disease and individual lifestyle. I most importantly had to learn the most effective, efficient, and caring way to communicate with patients, because this is what really matters in holistic healing: to send positive energy, to inspire them to initiate healing, to encourage them to practice therapeutic exercise, eat healthy, and to empower them to take charge of their life.

In my patient care, I design a healing plan for each patient. In western medicine, we use medication very often for symptoms, but not for cure. For example, many take a pain killer to relieve pain but don't know what is causing the pain. When I saw a patient suffering from pain, I would first find out what is causing the pain, then treat the cause. For example, headaches can have so many different reasons: stress, eye problem, neck problem, stomach problem, food allergy, back problem, nervous problem, sleeping problem, drug interaction, substance abuse, sensitivity to alcohol, brain tumor, the list goes on. Taking a pain killer without finding the cause, the patient would have a Yo-Yo effect: sometimes better, some times worse, up and down.

The healing plan I make for an individual patient includes: modifying their diet, their lifestyle, their mindset, and therapeutic Qi Gong exercises explicitly targeted to their illness. The results are amazing, and they did not even believe it was real. I also teach them Daoist philosophy and Daoist wisdom, which helps a great deal in removing their stress and relaxing their mind and body. By practicing these holistic methods, their quality of life is dramatically improved. When life quality improves, their health improves.

Since Chinese medicine theory is not easy to explain nor easy to understand, I often had to explain to patients using western medicine theory, then blended with TCM. It worked, patients did understand better, and they were more convinced. People come to me with all kinds of medical problems: heart disease, hypertension, digestive disease, hormonal problem, emotional and psychological issues, back problems, neck problem, frozen shoulders, cancer, liver disease, an endocrine disorder, women's issues, cancer, spiritual and mental issues, and much more. Some people were not feeling well for a long time, but their doctor could not find anything wrong, they then found they did very well with eastern medicine. I also helped many children with immune system problems, emotional problems, and behavior problems.

I have always been interested in the autonomic nervous system and focusing on regulating the autonomic nervous system, which plays a significant role in disease prevention and healing. That is my specialty, and not many know how to do this. I learned from both eastern and western medicine and by combining both eastern and western medicine and using it in my healing work. I integrate energy medicine, movement medicine, nutrition medicine, and Daoist healing wisdom in patient care and have achieved excellent results in physical, psychological, emotional, and spiritual aspects.

Considering the full range of illnesses that I had successfully treated, some medical doctors were curious and invited me to give a talk to explain how/why my methods were so effective. One pediatrician could not believe his patient's X-Rays were dramatically improved after my care. I had to explain how it worked in theory with both eastern and western medicine.

Among my patients, some were referrals from medical doctors, and some were referrals from patients, some were family members of my patients, some were friends of my patients, some were referrals from other holistic practitioners. I was so busy; it got to the point where I had to hire other practitioners. That was when my business was booming. I was twice on Boston TV (channel ABC, NBC), over ten times in different newspapers, many other times in various magazines. I am even featured in an exhibit on herbal medicine in the Boston Museum of Science. Some of my patients saw the photo of me in the Boston Museum of Science and were astonishing to know I was so "famous." But fame is not my intention; helping people to heal is my intention.

Since incorporating Qi Gong, Tai Chi, and other therapeutic exercise makes a big difference in healing, I wanted to know more, and I wanted to be able to explain to patients and students why these things work, and how they work. Every year, sometimes every other year, I went back to China to study Qi Gong, Ta Chi, and other martial arts such as Ba Gua Zhang and Xin Yi, from different teachers and world-famous masters. I just wanted to understand the healing effect of these martial arts. I also wanted to know if there were any side effects or restrictions when using these exercises and martial arts. I was fortunate to be mentored by Grand Master Feng Zhi Qiang, Professor and Master Li De Yin, Grand Master Zhu Tian Cai, Grand Master Duan Zhi Liang. Even though some of them had passed, they will be in my heart forever.

The more I learned, the more I was able to use both my medical knowledge and my Qi Gong knowledge to make connections between these exercises and body/mind/spirit.

Being busy with seeing patients, teaching evening classes, and providing certification training programs periodically, I was too busy and sometimes lost my patience: I was too quick to make decisions that led to adverse outcomes. Later, when I realized this, I consciously improved myself. I was more aware of my failings and continually trying to overcome them.

    A patient Marianne S. who was 19 years old, had lifelong depression. She was suicidal and had tried to cut herself several times. Medication did not work nor other therapies. Her mother took her to my office, hoping that I could help her. I was thinking, a suicidal young woman needs multi-angled healing, including Daoist teaching, herbal medicine, and body tune-up therapies (hands-on therapy). For a young schoolgirl, she probably cannot afford all this. So, I decided to take her home with me to work with her every day with no fee. She would stay in my house, eat with me, and I would provide insight and some therapies, all of these for free. One condition (I requested from her) was that she must not use any substance. She agreed. I intended to help her for two weeks; hopefully, she could be turned around and be able to choose the right path after that. I took her every place I went; people thought she was my daughter. I tried to encourage her to do more positive activities, things she liked to do, asked her to read daily, exercise daily, singing daily (she wanted to sing). Things were going well, and she was very happy for the first week. One day after the first week, she told me she used marijuana. That was like a big thunderbolt; I was so mad, I shouted with my anger. I said, "we had a deal not to use any substance, but you broke our agreement." I told her she had to leave my house after breaking her word. She cried, and we both cried, we hugged each other. I felt like a failure; I could not help her no matter how hard I tried. I doubted my ability to help others; I thought I was doing the right thing. I was somewhat angry at myself that I did not have an effective way of getting through to this young girl. When her family came to pick her up, we hugged again and cried again; yes, I cared about her and would certainly miss her. After this instance, I decided not to do this kind of volunteer work anymore. But from this, I realized that I was not patient enough, too quick to make a decision, and lost my temper, which is not the right way to be in my occupation.

    Several years later, she sent me a beautiful letter stated how much she appreciated the time with me, how much she thanked me for teaching her and helping her find her healing path. She told me she started to support herself and was doing very well after spending time with me. I then realized I did do some good after all.

Healing and recovering are two different things. Healing is to restore the person's health physically and to restore an emotional balance and improve the person's quality of life. Recovery is to allow the injured body parts/tissues to recover to normal function. If you had a cut, your damaged skin would recover in few days to a week; if you had a surgery, your recovery might take a few months to a year depending on the type of the operation. Some injury may not recover well because it didn't heal due to various reasons: stress, poor diet, negative mindset, emotional imbalance, poor sleeping, poor relationships, etc.

I had a patient Lisa who had lifelong depression. When she came to see me, she had pancreatic cancer and had undergone western treatment, including chemotherapy. I wanted to not only help her immune system but also to help her to restore her emotional balance. When she felt better, she wanted to move to another state, which I felt was not the right choice, because her emotion was still not balanced; it could cause the cancer to relapse. She moved out of the state anyway, far away from her parents. Within a year, she passed away.

Healing is holistic, and it involves the total body, mind, and emotion. It means to address the whole person.

Besides my healing and prevention work, I started to write books, by trying to write down all my experiences from my work, from being with people, from helping solve problems, what worked and what did not work, and lessons from teaching and observing. My first book, "Natural Healing with Qi Gong," was published in 2004; some years later, numerous other books of mine were published. One of my books, "Simple Chinese Medicine," got a Best Book Award, won third place in the Alternative Medicine category. I could not believe this because English is my second language, and I never expected to win anything, but I just wanted to teach people through my writing. Years later, three of my other books were up for Best Book Awards in different categories. My books went all over the United States in bookstores and libraries, also sold in different countries (English speaking countries). Sometimes I got calls or emails from people in different parts of the US as well as other countries. They had questions after reading my books and would like to learn more. Yes, this made my life busier, but it encouraged me to continue my writing. I was thinking: if I can be an award-winning author, I must have done something right, either people liked my books, or they liked my information, or they like my style. This year, in 2019, my book "True Wellness" (co-authored with another western doctor) won two awards. I am thrilled and grateful to have such a good friend and doctor to write together with me.

Since I had been doing some public speaking in my training courses and lecturing, I wanted to improve my speaking skills. In 2009, I joined the National Speaker Association (NSA). Every month I would go to a meeting where the organization invited well-known speakers to give a talk. I learned so much from each speaker, and this improved my speaking skills and speaking quality. The quality of my training programs got better each year. I learned how to add humor to my speaking, learned to make positive comments, and avoid negatives, like blaming. I learned to craft/prepare my speech, being careful not to offend anyone, regardless of their behavior or lifestyle. I am grateful for what I have gained, learned, and thankful to people I worked with, people I learned from, and friends and family who supported me.

In my first ten years, I worked very hard and learned as much as I could. In my 2nd ten years, I built on my success. Now, in my 3rd ten years, I cut back on my work and began to focus on my writing and educating.

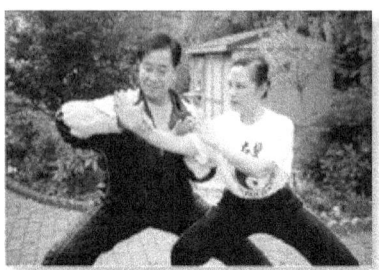 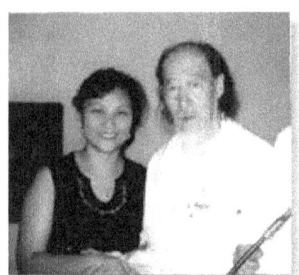

1. Master Zhu Tiancai from Chenjiagou
2. Grand Master Duan Zhiliang, from Beijing

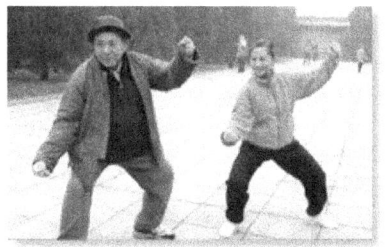 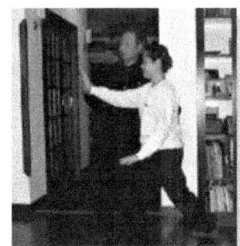

3. Grand Master Feng Zhiqiang, Beijing
4. Master/professor Li Deyin, Beijing

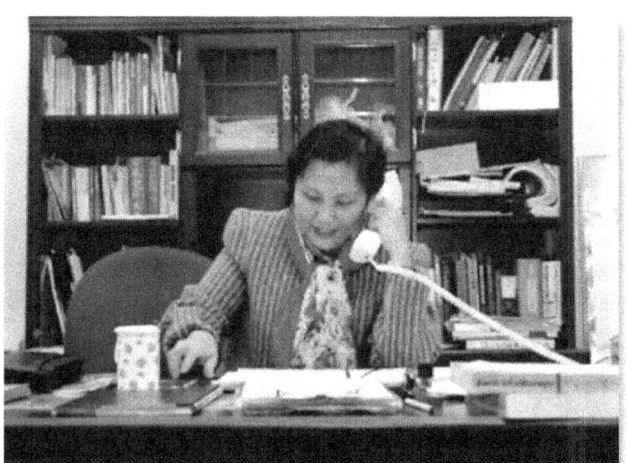

5. Patient consultation, Holliston, MA

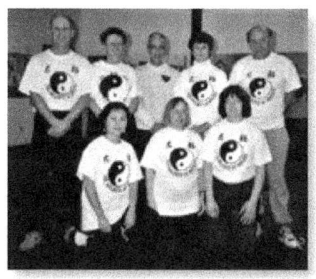 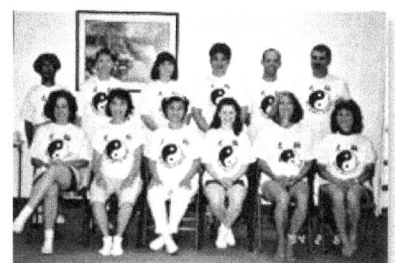

6, 7.. Teacher Training Courses

Chapter 13: Non-Profit Work

In 1998, I started an organization called: "Tai Chi & Qi Gong Healing Institute." I intended to gather likeminded people to study ancient Chinese philosophy (the Dao Te Ching), to practice Tai Chi and Qi Gong outdoors in nature, and to use Daoist philosophy to help people reduce stress and enrich their life and work. I believe with Daoist philosophy and wisdom, happiness can be maintained, and the quality of life can be improved. I have benefited from studying Daoist philosophy myself, and I wanted to continue to study in a group setting. The Dao provides a high standard for personal improvement in all aspects: physical, emotional, spiritual, life, relationship, career, fulfillment, and happiness.

In 2001, our institute became a non-profit organization (501C-3), which is a government-registered entity. Since the organization came into existence, we have been getting new members each year.

I have always felt that there is more to life than just making money, paying bills, raising children, buying stuff, and owning property. Life's deeper meaning is about understanding self, how to embrace positive energy, and understanding the connection between humans and the universe.

Human existence has two parts: a material part and a spiritual part. The spiritual part is not about religion nor obsessive personal beliefs. The spiritual part of life is about the higher power of self, the meaning of self, and self-exploration. Studying Tai Chi, Qi Gong, and combining the study of the Dao, helps people discover the power of their spiritual self. Daoist wisdom guides people to use material wisely, not excessively, and examine their spiritual life effectively. These teachings help the person to efficiently do things, living with less stress and free from negative emotional battles.

Our existence is not just about me, mine, my own; our presence can blossom by contributing, creating, giving, and helping others. What if we all care for each other, do things for each other, and help each other? What if we all live in a harmonious society with no hate, no stealing, no killing, no fighting, with abundant loving and nourishing? The commercial world may prevent us from achieving this. But we, humans, the most powerful beings, can change this, and we don't have to be controlled by the commercial world. We are the only ones who can create a harmonious world if we want to.

I remembered a while ago; I was living in Milford, Massachusetts. My husband and I were walking around our neighborhood. Somehow, we accidentally walked into a big field

and did not know it was private property. A man came out yelling and shouting at us "Please get off my property, this is my property." We tried to explain we live nearby, we are neighbors, and enjoyed the nature walk but did not know this was private property. He didn't care about our explanation. He continued to shout: "get off of my property, don't do this again." At that time, I was determined to put this story in my book, not because I was angry at him, nor to place blame. I wanted to share with my readers how I felt: some people are not as friendly as I thought, (Americans have a reputation for being friendly), especially neighbors. But even being friendly, maybe some people still have a lot of fear. But what is the quality of life if you carry so much fear in your life? You may say, "we have to be cautious not allow strangers to come into our yard." Yes, you are right, especially nowadays. I gradually got used to this, and understand why so many people have fear. But at that time, I was still comparing everything with the culture in China. We were always friendly with our neighbors, visited with neighbors, and helped each other in the neighborhood. I assume that it is different now.

Our organization had many meaningful activities. We organized a local event to join the world for World Tai Chi Day every year. After the 911 horrific instance, NYC had suffered a great deal; we went to New York Central Park, did Tai Chi, and Qi Gong in

Central Park. We had monthly activities such as hiking, camping, city walk, visiting different places, and monthly Daoist study meetings. Every year, we put on a natural healing conference, to educate people about how self-healing methodologies work, including how to integrate conventional medicine and holistic medicine in our health care, living with emotional freedom, nutrition, best practices for anti-aging, and boosting the immune system with Qi practice. Through the healing conference, we teach people how to balance energy, immune function, and provide healing tools that they can use to help themselves daily.

With all of these activities, our members develop friendships, gain strength from the group, and learn from each other. I do this totally as a volunteer. There is no financial gain, but I am rewarded by seeing so many people benefit from the organization.

I do this for myself too. I had many struggles in the past, but I gain so much wisdom from practicing and studying Daoist philosophy, practicing and teaching Tai Chi and Qi Gong. The Dao has helped me so much, enabled me to see things from a wider angle, to deeply understand natural patterns and the relationship between nature and humans. The Dao teaches me how to let go of the past, how to move forward with my life. How to gain strength for reaching my goals, and how to go with the natural flow. The Dao teaches me to be humble, to be thoughtful, to be more tolerant and patient, and to teach by example. From all these years of studying and practicing the Dao, I have become more relaxed, calmer, inward-thinking, and humble. I don't let myself get upset by stressful things that happen in my life. My mood and emotion have become even and balanced, and I'm able to handle many unexpected things that happened. The Dao also helped my relationship with my family, friends, people who worked for me, and people I had to deal with in business. The Dao is a kind of guidebook for living, a school of philosophy that can benefit every human being. Unfortunately, many people don't know this, which is another reason why our organization needs to exist.

What is "The Dao"?

Many times, people asked me what the Dao is. The Dao, officially called "Dao De Jing" in Chinese, was spelled Tao Te Ching in English, that is because most immigrants in early centuries who came to the United States were Cantonese (from Guang Dong Provence in China), and their language sound (dialect) is very different from the sound of mandarin. The Dao is an ancient Chinese philosophy that describes the absolute principle underlying the universe. It combines the principles of Yin and Yang and signifies the "way" or code of behavior that is in harmony with the natural order. The Dao is a natural phenomenon and spontaneous happening that cannot be named or described, nor twisted. The Dao is living wisdom, the methods, and the guide. The Dao is the intelligence of human behavior and the Way. You win if you go with the flow of the Dao, and likewise, the opposite is true, you would have more problems if you go against the flow of the Dao.

The Dao emphasizes searching for the world of perfect self without perfection. (In Japanese, like the concept of "Wabi-sabi.") The Dao helps seekers to find true self and inner peace and to allow the inner world to create a map with a beautiful path for themselves. Following along that beautiful path, they reach for the highest peak and illumination. When that comes, the chaotic world cannot destroy them, nor harm them. The Dao helped me to get through every kind of turbulence in life, kept me from insanity. The Dao teaches me to become a better person, a better leader, a better wife, a better mother, and a better teacher. The Dao helped me to always work on my weaknesses and to improve; therefore, my life became more comfortable, happier, and lighter. Members of the Tai Chi & Qi Gong Healing Institute have had similar experiences and greatly benefited from studying the Dao philosophy.

The Dao teaches us, "Keep it Simple." To practice the "simple," we start with the simplicity of our mind. Our mind is too busy, too complicated; we think too much, and many times that thinking is going in circles, which is not useful. When we simplify our mind, we can think more clearly. We speak intelligently, we do things efficiently, and we live without stress. These practices are a personal choice, and it is not about right or wrong: "less" versus "more," "I need," versus "I want," "material riches," versus "spiritual riches."

The Dao teaches us to be humble, genuine, peaceful, maintain good health, keep a harmonious and balanced life; it teaches us to focus, relax, to try not to try (wu wei), be pure and grounded, soft, yielding, flexible, moral, non-judgmental, clear-minded, observant, and positive. It values non-attachment, self-cultivation, unity, non-violent living, calmness, wholesomeness, and constant improvement of personal demeanor. With this kind of practice, you earn people's trust, earn a reputation, you can succeed, and you may have many friends.

The Dao is the opposite of pollution, toxins, violence, bragging, boasting, narcissism, anger, demanding, showing off, controlling, illness, turbulence, killing (weapons and words), pity, greed, selfishness, stubbornness, close-minded, divided, hating, teaching with empty words, egocentric, rigid, etc. The downside of living against the Dao is that you may have fewer friends, may have difficulty to succeed or reach your dream, you may have trouble maintaining a relationship, and may not have true happiness. But our brain and mind are very powerful and capable, and if you want to make any change, you can always make things better.

Our modern world provides us with an abundance more than what we need, but I cannot believe so many people still have fear. Maybe we don't have freedom even though we live in the country with the slogan of "Freedom for all"; perhaps we have seen too many negative instances, maybe we are not secured financially, physically, and emotionally; I don't know where all the fear comes from.

Many years ago, about two or three weeks before our annual natural healing conference, a girl named Robin, who was working for me (lovely girl) at that time, got anxious for not having enough people register for our conference. I kept telling her everything would be fine and told her there was no need to worry. She could not believe me. Then we had an unforgettable conversation:

> Robin: Dr. Kuhn, do you have fear?
> Me: No, I don't have any fear.
> Robin: What if you get sick?
> Me: If I got sick, I either see a doctor or help myself.
> Robin: What if you lose your job?
> Me: If I lose my job, I will find another one.
> Robin: What if your business doesn't do well?
> Me: If my business doesn't do well, I will work harder, try to find a way to make the business better.
> Robin: What if you cannot pay for your house?
> Me: If I cannot pay for my house, I would live in an apartment; if I cannot afford a big apartment, I would live in a small apartment; if I cannot afford to live in a small apartment, I would share an apartment with someone. Remember, there is always some way.
> Robin: What if a family member got sick?
> Me: If my family member is sick, I either take them to the doctor, or I will help them myself.
> Robin: What if your family member is severely sick, no one can help?
> Me: When that happens, I will still try my best because sometimes a miracle happens, and I have seen many miracles from my patient care. I will also pray for miracles.
> Robin: What if you are experiencing a disaster such as a hurricane, volcano, earthquake, you lose everything?
> Me: I hope it doesn't happen often. If this happens, I will rebuild my life step by step.

Finally, she gave up asking me questions because she knew I would have an answer for her every item. She then said to me with a sense of humor: you are not human, but I adore you.

I believe that after this conversation, she felt better and more relaxed. When the conference time arrived, we had more registered attendees than we expected. She then said to me, "Dr. Kuhn, you were right"! We had a big laugh.

Qi and the Dao:

The Dao and Qi go together. If you practice the Dao, your Qi most likely moves smoothly in your body; if you practice Qi (through Qi Gong, Tai Chi), your intuitive part of your brain improves, and you most likely are able to figure things out: what flows, what doesn't flow; what is right, what is not right. When you have the flow, your health is maintained; when you don't have the flow or are against the flow, illness develops. Thinking about it: when we are happy, our energy is good because our Qi flow is smooth; we feel comfortable, relaxed, and we want to do things. When we are unhappy or angry, our energy is low or imbalanced. We feel rage because our Qi is stuck; we feel uncomfortable, more tension in our body, more stress in our mind, and we have no interest in doing things, or we do wrong things. That is when we make mistakes, some people end up in jail. If the unhappiness lasts for a long time, we feel sick and maybe get a diagnosis of depression, anxiety, panic, migraine, insomnia, low libido, arrhythmia, Chron's disease, diabetes, hypertension, etc.

"Qi Gong" is not as some people think, "mysterious," or "superstitious." Some people mix up "Qi Gong" with "Fa Long Gong," which is a "cult" type practice, an obsessive practice using the Qi Gong name to do things for their purpose; it is a de-railed form of Qi Gong. Some Qi Gong forms can mislead people, then people may experience chaotic Qi, imbalanced Qi, and deviated Qi. Sometimes this is because of the teacher, or from improper teachings bordering on delusion.

Some people don't believe Qi Gong works because their doctor said it doesn't. Some doctors have even said the results are co-incidental and refuse to learn the theory of how Qi Gong assists in healing. Qi Gong has nothing to do with religion or politics; it's purely a form of exercise practice that involves our physical movement, mental focus, and deep breathing. In my book "Natural Healing with Qi Gong," it is explained in detail.

Some people say, "It is all in your head." Yes, it is in my head that I want to feel better and improve my health. With that "mindset," I initiate my action, and then with my practice, my illness disappears. No matter what you believe or don't believe, all that matters is that people feel better, they are happier, and they succeed in their career and life with the help of Qi and Dao practice.

Qi Gong practice involves total relaxation in the body, together with exercise movements that produce tremendous healing results. Westerners can understand "meditation," Qi Gong, and Tai Chi is "moving meditation." Being trained in both western medicine and traditional Chinese medicine, I see the correlations between the two types of medicine: meridian pathways and nerve pathways, organ energy and organ function, mind-body and Jing, Qi, and Shen are all comparable. I see the connection between anatomy and how Qi Gong is effective in healing. That is why I can explain Qi Gong healing using common western terminology, making it much easier for people to understand.

Qi Gong is a type of inward practice. Many people only pay attention to the external body and train with an external focus. Without inner practice, the external practice cannot be called Qi Gong. I had a person email me who claimed to have been trained by a big-name master in several forms of Qi Gong, but his email was filled with anger because I did not give the answer he was expecting. He even had a tone of prejudice against immigrants. He was surely not practicing correctly; he had not even learned the fundamentals of Qi Gong, regardless of how big the masters he had learned from were.

Qi practice teaches people to embrace peace, embrace the differences, and embrace our health in all aspects: mind, body, spirit, and emotion.

Daoist Practice:
Daoist practice has two parts: a philosophical part and a religious part. In China, Daoism is sometimes practiced religiously in temples. However, most practitioners all over the world focus on the reflective side of Daoism. This philosophical side is the area that our organization Tai Chi & Qi Gong Healing Institute focuses on.

Here are some chapters from the Dao De Jing
(Tao Te Ching: A New Approach, written by Jerry Dalton)

Recognizing Dualities (Chapter 2)
When all people know beauty as beauty, ugliness arises.
When all people know good as good, evil arises.
Thus being and non-being generate each other.
Difficult and easy complement each other.
Long and short form each other.
High and low support each other.
Tone and voice harmonize each other.
Front and back follow each other.

Therefore the sage:
Manages affairs without action,
Teaches without speech,
All things arise but he doesn't originate them.
He works without exception,
Accomplishes without taking credit.
Because he takes no credit,
The credit remains with him.

Self-Effacement, Self-Enhancement (Chapter 7)

The universe is eternal.
Why is the universe eternal?
It does not live for itself,
Thus it is everlasting.

Therefore the sage takes the hindmost,
And emerges foremost.
He effaces himself,
And is one with all.
Because he desires nothing,
He has everything.

Excellence and Non-Contention (Chapter 8)

The highest excellence is like water.
Water excels in benefiting all beings without contending.
It stays in places that men reject,
And therefore is close to the Tao.
The excellence of a dwelling is in its location.
The excellence of the mind is in its depth.
The excellence in giving is in being like heaven
The excellence in speech is in truth.
The excellence in leadership is in order.
The excellence in work is in competence.
The excellence in action is in timing.
He who does not contend will be free from blame.

Avoiding Excess (Chapter 9)

Better to stop in time than to overfill a vessel.
Over sharpen a blade and it will soon lose its edge.
A store of gold and jade cannot be protected.
Pride in wealth and rank brings calamity on oneself.
Withdraw when the work is done.
This is the Tao of heaven.

Developing Through Discipline (Chapter 10)

In embracing the one with body and soul,
Can you be undivided?
In controlling your vital breath,
Can you be supple as a newborn child?
In cleansing your inner vision,
Can you make it flawless?
Can you love and lead the people, without cunning?
In opening and closing the gateway to heaven,
Can you be like the female?
In seeing all things clearly,
Can you be without erudition?

Bearing and nourishing,
Bearing without possessing,
Rearing without ruling,
This is the mystic virtue.

Mystical Masters (Chapter 15)

The ancient masters were mystics with profound intuitive insight.
They were beyond understanding.
Because their subtlety could not be understood,
We can only describe their manifestations.
Cautious, as if crossing a wintry stream.
Hesitant, as if aware of danger.
Reserved, like a guest.
Yielding, like ice melting.
Simple, like an uncarved block.
Opaque, like muddy water,
Open, like a valley.

Muddy water, when stilled, gradually clears.
Something at rest, when moved, gradually comes alive.
Those who preserve the Tao, desire not to be full.
Since they are not full they can be depleted and yet renewed.

Small in Desire, Great in Action (Chapter 34)

The Tao is pervasive, flowing on the left and on the right.
It works and completes its affairs but never lays claim.
All things return to it but it never acts as master.
Ever desireless it is small.
All things return to it, but it never acts as master.
It is great.
Therefore the sage can accomplish great things,
Because he does not attempt to be great,
And therefore is truly great.

On Unity (Chapter 39)

These things from ancient times achieved unity:
Heaven achieved it, and became clear,
Earth achieved it, and became stable,
Spirit achieved it, and became sanctified,
The valley achieved it, and became full.
Leaders achieved it, and became statesman.
All of this resulted from unity.
Heaven without clarity would soon split apart.
Earth without stability would soon quake.
Spirit without sanctity would soon wither and die.
The valley without fullness would soon run dry.
Leaders without statesmanship would soon fall from power.

Therefore power is based on humility,
The low is the foundation for the high.
Because of this leaders call themselves alone, lonely, and unworthy.
Does this not acknowledge humility as a base?

The value of a chariot depends on the unity of its pieces.
Desire not to be as rare as jade,
Rather be as firm and as strong as rocks.

Riches and Fame, Self and Contentment (Chapter 44)
Which is more important, fame or self?
Which is more valuable, self or wealth?
Which is more painful, profit or loss?
Strong desires lead to wasteful spending.
Excessive hoarding leads to heavy loss.
To know contentment, is to avoid disgrace.
To know when to stop, is to avoid danger.
Thus one can endure for a long time.

Loss in Disorder, Gain in Nonaction (Chapter 57)
Govern a country with justice.
Wage war with surprise tactics.
Win the World by leaving it alone.
How do I know this is so?
By this:
The more restrictions there are, the poorer people become.
The more weapons there are, the more disordered the nation becomes.
The more knowledge and skill there are, the more strange novelties appear.
The more laws and regulations there are, the more thieves appear.
Therefore the sage says:
I take no action and the people reform,
I love quiet and the people become upright,
I do not meddle and the people prosper,
I desire not to desire and the people simplify their lives.

This is just a sample of the Dao De Jing. There are many interpretive works of literature you can find in libraries and book stores. They can be about Daoist practice, Daoist verses, or Daoist healing. The Dao De Jing was originally compiled in Chinese some 2500 years ago, so there are many different and interesting interpretations.

Our modern world is very far from Daoist views, and it may never get them back. We are too complicated, too creative, and don't know when to stop. We have too many new things coming into the world market every day and are overloaded with games, gadgets, and too much of everything. With all these new technologies, we have lost our privacy and freedom; we have lost precious time from so often looking at our smartphone, commercial advertisements, news, thousands of stories, and many are nonsense. We have so many social media "friends," but how many real friends do we have? How often do we get together, share feelings, share love, share our thoughts, share food, share our life?

Our personal data is being collected every minute. Commercial interests know everything about us from our searching and purchasing patterns on the internet. The more we look and search, the more they take advantage of us. Is this "Freedom"? Do we have freedom? The more we have or own, the less time we have. Time is the most valuable thing we have in our life; when we lose it, it's lost forever because time cannot be retrieved. We need to make use of the time we have most happily and efficiently. This way, when we are ready to leave this earth, we can proudly say: I had a good time in my life, I have no regrets, I'm ready to go.

The more we have, the more problems we have too. We get scam phone calls all the time that makes us not want to answer our phone calls anymore. Remember how we used to be happy to receive calls from friends and family? Remember when we used to spend more time with our family at the dinner table and on the weekends? For the younger generation, some of them are disconnected. They know social media very well, and they use their fingers to "chat" through their smartphones all the time, including walking on the street and even while driving. It's no wonder we have so many accidents. But how good are their people skills or interpersonal skills?

It is hard to believe that some people commit suicide because of social media bullies. But what if we make some changes by joining a "physical" social group that is suitable for you? Wouldn't it be better than using a smartphone for social interaction all the time?

We have too many environmentally destructive projects and non-stop greediness: always wanting more, more possessions, and non-stop building. We don't know when to stop, how to stop, and there is less and less protected land left on the planet; subsequently, not many places are left for animals. But we still have some people who are genuinely devoted to protecting our world, our mother earth, and the natural habitats which provide us with oxygen and beauty. If we take a moment to think it over, how much does it cost to live? Some may say "there's never enough," others may say "I am satisfied with what I have"; some say "I want more, I want to invest and make more"; others say "I am pleased no matter how much I have." Some have achieved, and some have died after achieving and getting what they wanted. Some suffer from severe illness after having made their fortune. Many people feel happy with what they have, even though they don't have much "excess."

Happiness is not found by satisfying all your wants, because desire has no end; there is always something else you want or something you want to compete no matter how much you have. But what if we put our intention toward "What I can do for others"? "What can I do to help or make changes"? The energy is different; our kindness can bring more joy to both you and others. When you think this way, and when you give or help others without expectation of getting back, you increase the positive energy in your body, your mind, and your surroundings. That positive energy will do much more for you than you might expect.

The material world does bring you things you want, but it also blinds your eyes and clouds your thinking. Can you believe someone killed a person to get a pair of Niki shoes? Can you believe two people could argue over "who came first" at a buffet dinner? And the worst is that one human can kill another human because they are not the same. Can you believe there are still no sensible gun laws in the United States after so many instances of shooting and killing?

I still have a hard time understanding why so many are still using drugs even though they know that drugs have killed so many people of all different ages. Sometimes I think: maybe we need to have a moral education initiative start-up in our school system.

Medicine also becomes more and more stressful; pharmaceutical costs increase every year, to the point where many people cannot afford their medication. Doctors (some of them) become greedy, prescribing opioids to patients so that they can get paid a chunk of money while their patients suffer from addiction. Corporate greediness is even worse: spreading chemicals to our land and water; the food industry only thinks of their profit regardless of what is healthy and what is not. Health insurance is even worse, no matter how much profit they make, they still ask for more and more, and then not cover some necessary medical expense and tests that the patient needs. If money produces evil, this money is meaningless. I have seen the sea animals injured by boats, I have seen doctors push surgeries that patients don't need, I have seen salespeople rob people's money with their words, and I have seen innocent people suffering from greedy business people.

How can we improve all this? People we can. We can do better than this; we can do good business with our conscience, care for each other, and we can get profit, and not be greedy. Money cannot bring you true happiness. But we can be happy if we all work together and we live smarter. Whatever we do, we must first think for a moment: Is this good for my health? Will this bother my conscience? Will this hurt the environment? Is this good for the earth? Is this ethical and moral?

Business does drive the economy; some companies are lovely in both product quality and customer service; other companies are greedy and unethical. What if we all did business without violating our moral code?

We understand that things don't change quickly, but I hope (wish) the world in the future has less greed, less hate, less judgmental living, less "me, me, me" that we see all the time.

I will continue to lead our organization, do the best I can to continue our mission, continue my teaching, and continue to spread positive healing energy. If you wish to support, please join me to help to build a better and harmonious society. To become a member, please visit us on the web: www.taichihealing.org. Together, we can achieve.

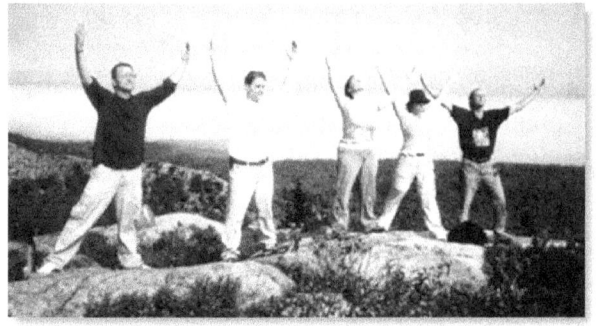

1. Practicing Qi Gong on top of a mountain, in Acadia National Park, Maine

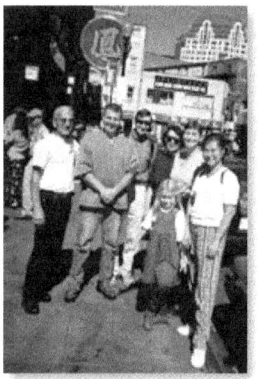 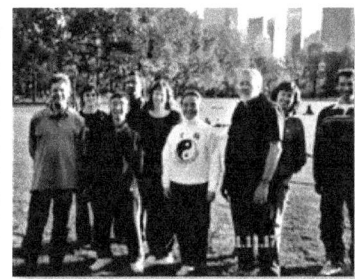

2. Chinatown in Boston
3. NY trip after 9/11, to support people in NYC

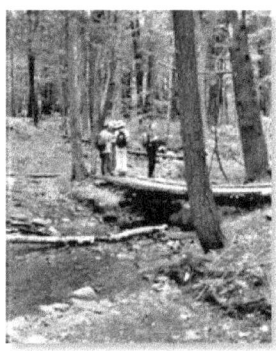 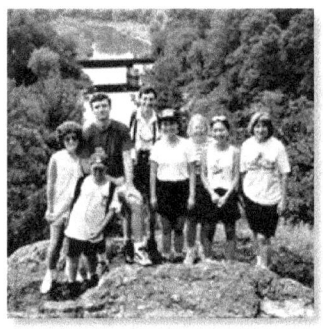

4. 5. Nature hikes

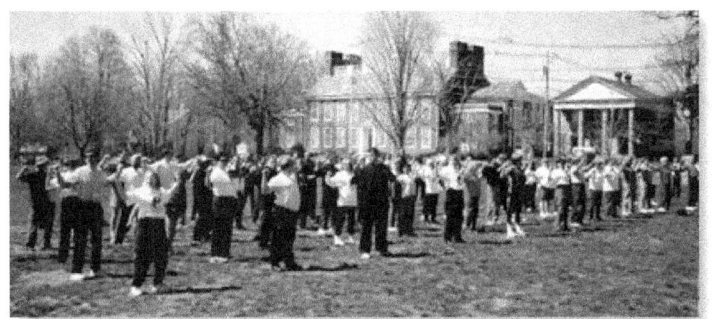

World Tia Chi Day, Framingham, MA

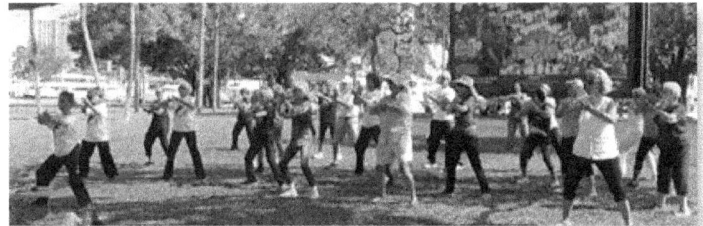

2018 World Tai Chi Day, leading practice Sarasota, FL

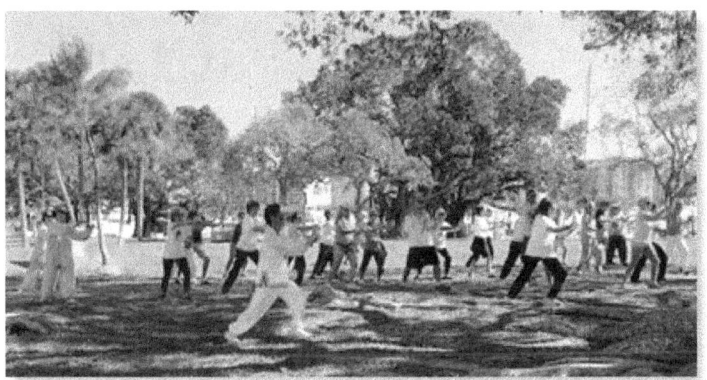

2019 World Tai Chi Day, lead group practice. Sarasota, FL

PART III: What I Learned and What I Gained

Chapter 14: Learning from Mistakes & Slip-ups

I have done many good things in my life, but I also have regrets. Hopefully, my reader, after reading my memoir, you may avoid some of my mistakes.

Life is a journey, not always a comfortable ride but a learning and a growing journey. No one is perfect, but through imperfection, we make the trip easier over time. Through mistakes we grow, we learn, we become wiser, and we succeed. In China, there was a sound support system with friends and family. If someone needed anything or needed some information, friends and family did their best to help. But in the US, I had to do everything myself, learn everything myself, and make every decision myself. It was not about good or bad. It was certainly not easy when you have to do everything yourself. I had to learn and grow from failure, mediocrity, striving until I succeeded. The good part is that I became stronger, gained ability through searching, learning, struggling, failing, and thriving.

I made some mistakes during those early days in the US. I had to manage my clinic, deal with patients, teach, and deal with the business. At first, I did not have the correct way to deal with difficult people. I did not deal well with criticism either. I was impatient, did not want to spend much time explaining things to patients, and I was a little arrogant. But later, I became better and better at it. I also made mistakes in my financial decision making; instead of keeping things simple, I made my work and life more complicated by expanding my practice, I was hot-headed. When you expend a business, you have more expenses, and it costs more to do business. Since I am not good with business matters, only good with my healing/teaching skill, I should not have expanded my business. I should be who I am and be content. Later, when I paid more attention to the essence of the Dao, I was able to turn things around and make corrections.

I was smart, talented, creative, fast reacting, intelligent, hard-working, eager to learn and to improve. But I was not wise. The first eight years, I was impatient, had a narrow view, had self-induced stress, made quick decisions, and I was not careful. I did not have adequate communication skills until later when I learned from professional speakers, taking some classes, reading numerous self-help books, and observing reactions from people, my students, my patients, and my audiences. I practiced awareness and put awareness into my life, my work, and my health. I consistently guided myself and reminded myself of Daoist wisdom and put it into my daily practice. I got better. Learning without practicing did not mean much; learning with practicing changed my life and my whole personality.

I remember, at one time, when I was offering a CEU program for nurses, I made a big mistake with my wrong use of words. I had over 25 people participating in the program. The topic of the program was "Chinese Medicine and Natural Healing." It was about healthy living and natural healing. One segment of my talk was about a healthy diet and maintaining a healthy weight. I accidentally said, "fat people" when talking about how to control weight. There was one nurse who was overweight; she sat in the last row in the room. In the afternoon session, I realized this nurse did not return to my class. I felt terrible; I regretted this and wished I could take my words back. People who have a weight issue may have a genetic reason, medical reason, emotional reason, too much stress, or medication, and so on. It is not their fault to have a weight problem. They need more help, and I should have had more sympathy, compassion, and been more considerate, especially with words and how to say things in a non-insulting way. From this experience, I started paying more attention to my talks, my speech, crafted my lectures and speaking. I tried to be more thoughtful and tried not to hurt anyone's feelings when speaking either to an individual or a group. Speaking in public, you cannot say things as in casual conversation, where you only want to have fun. When speaking in public, your speech needs to be considered and carefully crafted. Speakers should never hurt anyone's feelings nor have any bias in their remarks. I decided to learn more about how to develop a higher quality in my public speaking.

I joined the National Speakers Association in 2009. To join this organization, a prospective member needs to have specific qualifications. Since I had been teaching for so long, I had no problem joining. Each month the organization invited world-famous speakers to give a one-day lecture on a Saturday. There were all different topics and speaking techniques. I learned so much and then started using this knowledge in my teaching and speaking programs. I learned how to bring humor to my speaking, how to say things pleasantly, how to correct other's mistakes without criticizing. I learned to use positive words rather than negative comments and how to get the audience's attention. I also learned never to brag no matter what level I reached, not to talk about "Me," but rather to talk more about the positive "You." I set higher standards for myself; I told myself that I had to put in a 110% effort even if I could only do 100%. As I kept on learning, kept trying, kept improving, I could see myself become calmer, more balanced, and peaceful, and able to see things more clearly. My training programs did improve, and I got many high marks on my class evaluation forms.

In my patient care, I learned to be open-minded, listening to patients, paying attention to their physical needs and emotional needs, helping them to figure out the best way for their healing. I also paid attention to avoid being seen as "too commercial," even though our broader health care system has already turned into commercial care. I did not want to be like that. If my patients didn't need any herbs or supplements, I honestly told them that they didn't need them; but if they did need them for their medical problems, I would prescribe specific herbs or nutrition for their healing. Seeing my honesty, patients had more and more trust in me. That is how I got more and more patients to the point I had to hire other practitioners to help with the workload.

I tried to be available for patients, even if it was my day off. I remember at one time, a woman was in crisis, was crying, and desperately wanted to see me. I declined because it was my day off. Later I regretted this. When someone needed me, I should make myself available; it was my job to help people. Then, I made changes and was able to accommodate patients even on my day off as long as I was not far away from home.

Seeing that people were not getting better from other medical care, I developed holistic healing methods: multi dimensioned care: treatment, herbs, nutrition, exercise, diet, mind re-direction. It made a big difference.

I tried to practice honesty in everyday life. If patients were not improving as I expected, I would tell patients the truth that I could not help them anymore, or I would refer them to a doctor to get more tests or try other therapy. I tried not to criticize western medicine because western medicine has many useful methodologies that we need. I was able to guide patients on how to make the right choice in their conventional care. Honesty certainly earned my patient's trust.

Another mistake I made was that I rejected an invitation to give a free talk at Northeastern University (one of the departments related to health and wellness). The reason I declined their request was because I would have had to cancel all my patients that day (I was busy and had a lot of patients at that time), which may have led to losing a bit of money. Later I realized how stupid I was; I had a narrow mind and did not see the bigger picture. I regretted that for many years.

In the beginning, I was too rigid when talking about Chinese medicine, which is not easily understood. Later I tried to use a different way to explain and make sure I was not blaming western medicine, which I did previously. Both approaches to medicine have their value.

I also tried to respect other holistic practitioners. If the patient came to me from another holistic medicine office but wanted me to help them to improve, I would provide treatments to the patient to make her/him feel better, then ask the patient to go back to the original office to do their maintenance care. My job is to make patients feel better, not to try to get more patients to boost business. That also earned people's trust; I ended up getting more patients from referrals.

I learned to downsize, tried to avoid ego or showing off, tried to be humble, not loud, tried not to brag about myself, even though I got hundreds of letters from my patients and students thanking me for healing their illnesses; thanking me for helping them change their life, and thanking me for empowering them. After my books came out, my reputation got higher, especially after my book "Simple Chinese Medicine" got an award. I got more letters, emails, and phone calls from readers. Not only did they tell me how much they liked my book, but they also wanted appointments or phone consultation with me, which made my life busier, but I tried to keep a lowkey lifestyle.

One of my habits is living with a positive mindset. I tried to do things positively, teaching patients to practice being positive, and being positive when teaching students. This kind of teaching has changed many people's life. I did not want to take credit because it was them looking for me to help them; their initiative made the difference. If they remained angry and did nothing, they would not feel better.

I learned to be flexible, not so rigid. I was rigid before, which made other people nervous or afraid of me. I came from a military family. I grew up with strict teaching, then went through a chaotic early life during the cultural revolution in China. There were some rigid personality traits in me. But I always believe anything can change, and so I can change too. When I was more relaxed, soft, flexible, people around were more comfortable. I continued to improve my "people skills," and the more I progressed, the more I attracted people.

Writing in English is very challenging for me. No matter how many books I write or how many awards I get, I will never be as good as an English writer. But I firmly believe that I can improve every year as long as I continue to write. Reading English was not easy for me, either. I was always a slow reader partially because my eyes sometimes don't focus well. But I force myself to read, trying to overcome the difficulty. The more I read, the more relaxed I become. That again proves my point: anything can change.

I continue to work on my emotional and spiritual improvement, learn to balance life, to be with nature, try consciously not to let stress affect my life, and truly enjoy the freedom in my life.

Chapter 15: Learn to be a Good Leader

People often think that a leader is a boss, chairman, manager, CEO, principal, director, teacher, coach, president, etc. They believe leadership qualities only belong to these kinds of people. A leader is more than just a boss, executive, or CEO. Leadership is a quality of a person who shows leadership in any situation, such as problem-solving, dealing with people, softening a tough situation, having a pleasant demeanor in public and at home. Leadership can be exhibited by anyone who wants to reach a higher level of personal being. If you have a family, a good leader can create a happy and harmonious family; if you have a job, you show your ability of able to manage your stress; if you have a girlfriend or boyfriend, you can maintain your relationship with your words and action. I was not perfect, but yes, I tried my best to put family first on top of searching and exploring my path for many years. One good thing is that I always wanted to learn and improve. It shows in my ability to take criticism positively, which I could not do before.

I founded the organization "Tai Chi & Qi Gong Healing Institute," which also means I started to train myself to be a leader. I wanted to be a good leader, and I tried to lead by example; I wanted to help our members to achieve. Earlier, I did not have patience with callers; I was too quick, did not want to take time to explain things to callers. I was not patient with people who worked for me, either. I set high a standard for myself, but I should not have tried to put this high standard on other people. People who worked for me were good people, and I should be grateful. As long as they did their best, I should be grateful. Later I became better and changed my way of dealing with people, became passionate, and exhibited more kindness.

Over the years, I learned to appreciate everything in life, work, friendship, and relationships.

I appreciate all the help I got from friends, family; and I appreciate all the people who used to work for me and helped me in so many ways. I also learned from them too. Deborah K. was very pleasant to work with, she was the first secretary working in my office and also taught me how to drive a car with a standard shift; Paulette C. was a nurse who helped me start my CEU programs for nurses, she was very well-organized, smart, and efficient. Judy S. is such sweetheart also has a gentle soul, friendly, hardworking and pleasant to work with; Jeannie and Tom H are very kind and giving, so patient with people, and helped me in all aspects; Stacy F. was the first acupuncturist who worked in my office and had such an excellent way of talking to people and treating people; Steve S, was also acupuncturist has a most exceptional personality, friendly, and good sense of humor which everyone liked; Jeannie D. was the first person I trained and who then taught Qi Gong in my school for many years, was so gentle, sincere, punctual, and disciplined; Ann W. was indeed a sweetheart who also has a great sense of humor made me laugh every time we were together. Ellen M. was an excellent Qi Gong/Tai Chi teacher, is gentle, kind, thoughtful. Ann B. was also acupuncturist is very organized, detailed, and very good with record keeping. Martin L. was a Tui Na therapist, is very friendly, and has a gentle way of treating people; Deborah K was also Tui Na therapist, has such a soft and gentle way that people liked. Joe F. taught both Qi Gong and Tai Chi, good teacher, is sincere, kind, always helped me anytime I needed help. Deborah G. was also a Qi Gong teacher, is so gentle, kind, very thoughtful. Vickie S., my volunteer, so sweet, lovely, she helped with anything I needed. I had many excellent, diligent students who studied with me for many years. They also often helped me any time I needed anything. Each one of them are special and unique: Jim Agneta, Bob Mazzaires, Josee Arel, Kathleen Sakovitz, John Skillings, Deric Delfino, Miyo Yokota, Ellen Kirstein, Joyce Cerruti, Larry O'Sullivan James Gray, Elizabeth M., Marie Murphy, Shawn Amacost, JoAnn Jacobs, Carol J. Eric B. Cynthia Hansen, Marsha Wintringham, Alon B, Dorothy Vine, and many more. I may not spell their last name correctly, but I certainly appreciate their trust in me and supporting me and give me the courage to move forward.

I also had many student volunteers who proofread my books, gave me feedback, and write comments. I am so grateful to have so many beautiful people in my life helping me. Without these wonderful people, I could never accomplish my work, my mission, and my writing.

I do have my regret, but later became a lesson I learned. In the past 17 years owning my clinic/school in Massachusetts, I organized China trips and took students and patients to China 4 times. I intended to have them experience a different culture, learn something from the culture. One of the trips traveling in China involved taking an overnight train to another attraction. At that time (about 2002), the train car quality was not that comfortable, sleeping in a berth was better. There are soft berth and hard berth; the soft berths were in a separate room with four beds: two upper berths and two bottom berths, similar to bunk beds. The beds were a little wider than the hard berth (beds). Hard berths were not so private; Three beds on each side: top, middle, and bottom. Therefore, it allowed for six people sleeping. The hard berth had no privacy, six beds in a space, and beside the area is the walkway for public use. There were eight people on this trip, but we got only one soft berth with four beds: two upper beds and two lower beds, with a door you can close to keep privacy. The rest of the group were sleeping in a hard berth.

I did not think much about it but took a soft berth along with three others. Among the other three, there was a woman (I don't want to say her name) who had a mild form of MS, and her husband was also on this trip. I did not think to let her husband take the soft berth so that he could take care of her. After this trip, I so regretted my behavior, my selfishness, my carelessness. I criticize myself for not being a good trip leader. A leader should always put others first, yourself last, but I did not do that. Many years later, I heard that woman passed away, which made me feel even worse.

But I learned: to be more thoughtful, more careful, be selfless, give more.

Being the leader of a non-profit organization, "Tai Chi & Qi Gong Healing Institute," I am doing this as a volunteer. I put my time and energy to help members to improve their health, emotion, Qi, attitude, and skills for managing their stress. Since I did not do this for making money, to maintain this organization, I don't have pressure. I have lovely volunteers who are kind, loving, sincere, and having good morals. I am happy to be with them, and they are pleased to be with me too. It is a mutual connection of energy between our members and me. By doing this, I continue to learn and to grow.

Studying the Dao De Jing has helped me very much! The Dao enabled me to become a better leader, teaching me to be humble and giving, reminding me not to be stressed, guiding me to the right path, and showing me how to lead by example.

Chapter 16: Embrace and Cherish Cultural Differences

I hope this chapter does not offend anyone, which is not my intention. It is from my own experience of what I see, what I hear, and what I experienced. I share with readers my positive purpose.

One of the good parts of living in the United States is that you can experience many cultures. To experience different cultures is not about judging which culture is better; instead, it is about learning from the differences.

People do things in different ways, eat a different way, and sing songs in a different style or play music in different styles, and dress differently. From the differences, we learn from each other. For example, some of the designs on fabric from Japan, or Africa are so uniquely beautiful; some of the glass art from the middle east are so intricate and splendid. There is no such thing as a perfect culture or perfect people, but we are indeed all similar. Every culture is a unique culture. If we are open-minded, we can always learn something from other cultures.

Living in two different cultures, experiencing different people, I saw different ways of doing things, and I learned a lot. I was born and lived in China for 30 years, and lived in the United States for another 33 years. I have seen unique things in both countries. Trying not to be judgmental, here are some of my thoughts from my observations and experience. It may not be precisely accurate; it is only from my observations and impressions in general.

First of all, let's begin with the values of the two countries (in general, but not all):

American values: Independence, privacy, directness, equality, informality, competition, time and efficiency, work ethic, consumerism. For detailed explanations, please visit:

https://usahello.org/resources/american-values/

Chinese Values: The core value is harmony; around this harmony, everything works. "A peaceful family will prosper (jiahe wanshi xing, 家和万事兴)" is a famous and widely embraced saying. Harmony means "proper and balanced coordination between things" and encompasses rationale, propriety, and compatibility. Rationale refers to acting according to objective laws and truths. Propriety indicates suitability and appropriateness. The value of harmony advocates "harmony but not uniformity." Properly coordinating different things by bringing them together in the appropriate manner allows them to develop from an uncoordinated state to one of coordination, from asymmetry to symmetry; and from imbalance to balance. Modern Chinese society tries to maintain harmony between humankind and nature, between people and culture, between members of different communities, and between mind and body. Much of this comes from Confucius's teachings, Daoist living, and Buddhist practice.

For a detailed explanation, please visit: https://carnegietsinghua.org/2013/11/21/china-s-traditional-cultural-values-and-national-identity-pub-53613

People:

We all know that China has a vast population. There are so many people. And the Chinese people have so many particular traits. During any hard time I ever had in China, I got so much help from friends and family that certainly made my life easier. When my friends and family needed help, I helped them with my best effort. I felt lucky to have such good friends and family.

Generally speaking, Chinese people (the majority) are amiable, warm-hearted, giving, welcoming, selfless, and hard-working. In China, if we have friends, pretty much we have these friends for a lifetime, which explains why Chinese people cherish friendship so much. Friends like to get together periodically, to chat, to laugh, to share, and to help each other when in need. If you have very close friends, you can share your feelings with them and then get comfort from these good friends. Occasionally you miss judge and make lousy friends who may stab in your back and make you feel miserable. But you learn from this, and you become better at making good friends.

When friends get together, they can be loud in public places because they love to be lively, bustling. They don't care too much about privacy, and they like to share their thoughts, including personal drama. But it depends on the individual's personality; some people don't want to share.

In public places, people don't say hi if they don't know each other. If you try to say hi, they may think you are strange or think you may want to take advantage of them. When my son went to China 5 years ago trying to say hi to people, people looked at him did not know what to do with him: he is cute, handsome, friendly, but a stranger. Eventually, he learned the culture. I thought it was a sweet story.

Most people are content, satisfied, enjoy shopping, or window shopping (we say "guang jie") or stroll around the street. Even when my husband and I go back to China, we sometimes say, "Let's go guang jie." Younger people study hard, work hard, and now play hard too.

Living and working in the United States for 30 years, I feel lucky to say that I have met so many terrific people. Among them, there were my students, my patients, my volunteers, people who worked for me, people I knew from attending events or activities, people from different organizations, and some neighbors. They are kind, gentle, polite, sincere, resourceful, sincere, smart, loving, caring, and many of them were hard-working people.

In public, Americans tend to be careful not to be bothersome. They are polite, have good manners, and enjoy their privacy. Even when shopping, we often say hi to each other. I remember when I came to the US, I learned that in public places, it's "ladies first." I was so happy to see the respect for women; I felt like I came to a magical country.

Since American often relocate due to work, family, or whatever reason, sometimes it is not easy for newcomers to make friends. So, some newcomers may feel lonely. Eventually, they find a way to make friends. I felt lucky that I have met so many good people, good friends over 30 years.

You may notice this cultural behavior when meeting new Chinese people. If you have Chinese people come over for dinner, they may say, "I had enough," but actually, they are just being polite and don't want to take too much of the food. If you go to a Chinese home for dinner, and you praise their cooking and delicious meal, they will say, "No, I am not good." They want to be modest and polite, but they are happy to hear that. You may often hear from Chinese "I am not that good"; this does not mean they are not good; they are only trying to be polite and modest.

Food and dining:

For thousands of years, China has had one of the world's most marvelous culinary cultures. There are many different styles of cooking, and each province has its character of food flavor, diversity, and way of cooking. We all know that real Chinese food is delicious. We even enjoy some "noble attempts" at Chinese cuisine in US Chinese restaurants. The dishes are so creative and so thoughtfully crafted. There's so much variety and flavor that it has drawn people from all over the world. Chinese people love to eat, eat well, like variety, and especially enjoy the excellent taste. People love to get together to eat out and enjoy sharing the multiple dishes they order. They enjoy this kind of social gathering. They have a tradition of offering to pay for the meal, which makes them feel good to give, to provide. You may see Chinese people fighting to pay the bill in a Chinese restaurant. My husband could not understand this (he is an American). Chinese people don't like to appear "cheap"; nobody wants to be friends with a cheap person. Paying the bill is one of the good traits of Chinese people. If people did not get a chance to pay the bill this time, they would try hard next time.

There is always a variety of dishes in the restaurant, and many dishes are not high in calories, mainly vegetarian dishes. They do have delicious fried food too, but you don't eat those often.

Since the food in China is so flavorful, sometimes I feel like I want to go to China to eat and try every dish in the restaurant. Every time after visiting China, when I came back to the US, I would often look in the refrigerator and say to myself: what can I eat? I then realized that I had to learn to cook myself if I wanted to eat flavorful food.

America has diversified cuisine due to having immigrants from all over the world. Not only are there Western foods, such as French, Italian food, but also food styles from Mexico, the Middle East, Africa, China, and Vietnam, etc. Thank goodness for our multi-cultured country. The only thing is that there is somewhat of a loss of authenticity unless you try very hard to find genuine ethnic food. Many people try to eat different food from different styles of cooking, especially in the younger generation who are open-minded. Several things are different here: we usually order a dish we like for our self, and it's not often shared. That may be because some people have food allergies, or are picky eaters, or for other medical reasons. Some people are not willing to try new dishes, and they often order the same meal every time. Some recipes they like contain high calories and high fat but taste good, which may contribute to heart disease, hypertension, diabetes, obesity, high cholesterol, and many other conditions. One thing I noticed is that many people in the US have various digestive problems that I did not see in the Chinese population.

There have been many changes in American's diet and lifestyle in the past 20 years. Nowadays, younger people, professionals, and college students pay more attention to their diet, eating foods with low calories, fresh foods, more whole foods, proper nutrition, and a healthier home-cooked diet. The older generation does make changes in their diet and drinking habits mostly after something happens, such as a heart attack, diabetes, hypertension, or other disease. Some of them may make changes after seeing others suffer from those diseases or dying from those diseases. Healthy eating may also be related to one's education level too.

Education:

In China, people very much see education as the most crucial thing in bringing up children. In China, the school is not free, and parents have to pay money from kindergarten to college. It costs a lot of money to give a child a good education. Almost everything is about the child. Teachers are highly respected, and they do make a decent amount of money teaching and tutoring. If the child doesn't want to learn, the parents will put pressure on him and try to find any way they can to make him learn. They tell the child that they pay so much money for education; it would be a waste if he is not learning.

Not only do children study in school, but parents also pay extra to get tutors to make sure their child gets ahead of others. Many of the parents want their children to go to a school with a good name, a good reputation so that the child can find the best job after graduating from college or graduate school. After being hired, that child must work very hard because he/she wants the parents to be proud. The parents' intention is all for the child's future, but some kids may not always appreciate that. Most children understand their parents' efforts to improve their opportunity. Many children have minimal time to play, to do social activities, and to have fun, but in the long term, they will be doing fantastic work. The good part is that most children do follow through. In addition to the academic component, children may also be tutored in music, art, athletics, and so on. Many parents want their child to be a genius, which often may cause competition between parents. Some parents are arrogant about their child going to the right school, having good grades, and they love to brag about their child. When the child doesn't have good grades, some parents may feel embarrassed, sad, unable to show their faces in public. Some feel ashamed, but eventually, they realize each child has their individual gift, and the health of the child and good morals are all also important.

Not every family can afford all these tutors; therefore, the pressure on some families is very high. Sometimes the child may blame the teacher who charges so much money. But I did see one report that a child killed herself because she could not handle the burden that her parents had.

But some Chinese kids are spoiled, and they don't need to worry about tuition paid by their parents, and they may not care much about study either. One thing I have to say, no matter whether you have an education or no education, most Chinese people have a good work ethic; they work very hard and don't usually complain about working hard (in general).

Education is so different here in the US. The school is public, and it is free for all students from kindergarten to high school. Many programs offered in school are also free of charge, such as: after school programs such as art, music instruments, theater, and many different sports; free tutors for students who have trouble understanding the course; special ed for kids who have special needs; free public transportation if students live more than 2 miles (may differ by city or town). If parents think a school in another city or town is better, they are free to transfer their child to that school. All these educational benefits take away the burden from parents. The funding for public school comes from our taxes. But there is a reality here that many teachers don't make a good income. Living in a high-cost city or area, some of them had to change their careers.

The majority of students do well, but some children don't see that learning is essential. Sometimes we see on the TV or hear from friends who are teachers about abusive behavior in school, either teacher abuse student or student abuse teacher. Or students may bully each other. (This can never happen in China; school officials would punish any offender.) The level of respect for teachers is less here compared to China. The learning ambition of the students varies depending on the city, town, area, and the parent's education level. One thing that troubles me is that there is a drug problem in high school (also in college), and I don't understand why there is no solution in this country.

Here college students, like Chinese college students, some study hard, and others don't care much. The difference is that most students have to get a loan for some or all of their college tuition because of the enormous expense of college tuition that is not something many families can afford to pay in full. Some students are very stressed about their future if they can or cannot get a good job to pay off their loans. Student stress can be from expenses, test grades, lack of sleep, being unable to cope, depression, alcohol, relationships. Some of the pressure comes from technology, especially smartphones. Too often, some are using it 24/7. They use smartphones so much that it causes them to lose time to study and sleep. They get emotional stress from harmful information and being unable or having no time to do things they enjoy doing.

Similar to China, some have good work ethics, and others don't.

The difference in teaching, from my own experience, is the US education has more emphasis on independent thinking, which helps a great deal for students to gain skills for problem-solving, organizing, and independence. What I remember when I was in school, the teacher taught whatever the textbook said. I don't have much knowledge about Chinese education in school now. It may be the same as the US.

Overall, both countries have good parts and weak parts which can be improved if we open minds and are willing to learn from each other.

Choosing to live in the city

In the early years, most people in China lived in the town where they grew up, and where they worked. But in recent years things have changed so much, becoming very much westernized. People change jobs, relocate, and move to other cities. People want to live in a town where there is an excellent school system, better job opportunities and better pay, and a better environment. Even though the small city may have a better deal for housing, things cost less, and it's easier to find a job; some people still prefer to live in a bigger city where the education is better, and there is more of everything.

Here in the US, some people may like to be close to a better school; others look for a price they can afford, or a beautiful setting and environment, or a good deal such as a modest home with a big lot size. Some people choose to live in a house or apartment that is close to work, which makes a lot of sense: less stress commuting and saving precious time. Those may not always be the case, as I mentioned before; it's just my observation.

Buying a house (apartment):

In China, most working people lived in the city where there are only apartments for purchase (and a limited term of ownership). The land belongs to the government, but the apartment belongs to you after the purchase. Most people save money for a long time until they have enough to buy an apartment. If they don't have enough money, family members who have money will help them to buy the apartment. Now China has changed, similar to western culture, and has begun to offer mortgages. Even with that, people still want to pay as much as they can, to reduce the years of paying the mortgage or have a smaller monthly payment. This way, their stress is lower. The apartment can be 2 to 4 bedrooms, from 75 to 150 square meters, with a balcony which is mostly used for hanging clothes or keeping some potted plants. Things have changed so much since I left; even younger people working very hard cannot afford to buy an apartment, especially in bigger cities. Many of them can't afford to buy an apartment until they get older when they have more money. Housing is so expensive, many young people just rent, and some share a flat with roommates.

Here in the US, it seems that anyone can buy a house. The mortgage system is very accessible, and people may make a small down payment, then pay their mortgage each month. Banks make a lot of money from mortgages. Unfortunately for people, there is always the risk of losing their job, and losing their house, it puts a lot of stress on people. I am not sure, but I think many people have a competitive mind: if you can buy a house, then I should be able to buy a house. That benefits the banks. If I did it again from the beginning, I would prefer saving until I had enough before I buy a house, or enough to pay an 80% down payment. I would feel much more relaxed.

Raising Children:

I think raising children is one of the most challenging things for Chinese parents living in the United States. In China, generally speaking, children obey their parents, respect their parents; they understand parents have the best intentions for them. If parents pay thousands of dollars for a child to take piano lessons, the child will study, will practice, and will become an excellent piano player. You may have already seen many Chinese musicians on the world's stages. Some of them may also have a good job but still play well with their instruments. There is absolutely no drug issue in school; if you use drugs, you go to jail, without exception. If you sell drugs, you may get the death penalty.

Maybe the situation is different now, but as I remember, I always respected my parents, always wanted to please my parents, and do whatever my parents asked me to do. All my sisters and brothers did the same thing. I still think this way: they gave me life, taught me how to live my life, I should be grateful, thankful, and respectful to them.

Chinese children who are born and grow up in the United States are not the same as kids in China. They have to deal with peer pressure; get influenced by American culture (mainly from kids in school) some good and some bad. The good part is that they learn to be independent both in life, academic study, and not afraid of trying things. The bad things are drug issues, girl issues, stealing medications from parents, alcohol abuse, sex issues, bullying issues, some are obnoxious. At home, they talk back, sometimes yelling at parents, disobeying parents, then they tell parents, "You need to learn." Even though, to some extent, it is true the parents need to learn, this should not be said by children (at least not in Chinese culture). But it is a new culture, and it is tough for some Chinese parents to accept children talking back like that. It is difficult for both children and parents. As I remember, both of my children got bullied in their school. When my daughter got bullied on the school bus, she cried when she came home. With anger to know my daughter got bullied, I immediately called the school and explained the situation. The next day my daughter told me the principle announced in school that it is not allowed to bully anyone, which made me feel better. But my son got bullied and did not tell me; when I found out later, I asked him, "what did you do to defend yourself?" He said, "I just ran away." I felt terrible, and then I started to teach him some martial art, and later in high school, I send him to China to study martial art such as Xin Yi, Shaoling, push hands, Sanda, etc. Even now my son is a grown man, I still ask him to study martial art, not for fighting, but for internal strength that can help everything.

I was bullied when I was young; I was also insulted when I was older. But nothing can affect me anymore because I have internal strength. My inner strength came from practicing Tai Chi, Xing Yi, Qi Gong, and studying Daoist philosophy. But during those years raising children, my internal strength was not high enough to teach them. Hopefully, from these life experiences, they will grow stronger and gain more abilities and be able to handle and deal with life in this world.

Rating for success:

For many years, the Chinese always believed that if you have money, that means you are successful. Even some people with no education but doing business got lucky; they were considered "successful." Then the consequence of having money was to buy a big house, a bigger car, brand-name consumer goods, just like here in the US. They wanted to show how successful they are and were proud to be rich. Some people are humble, successful but not showing off. One time when I was living in Boston, I had a friend who visited me from China. She asked me to guess how much money she paid for her pants. I said 100 to 150 yuan ($15 to 20 US dollars). But she told me that she paid 1000.00 yuan these for pants, which is $155.00 US dollars. I would never pay that much for a pair of pants, not because I cannot afford, but because I don't think it is necessary.

Chinese people do judge others by looking at their clothes, shoes, what they do, what their parents do, etc. That has been going on for thousands of years, and it may take time to change. But I think it is getting better, and many people who came from a low-income family do become very successful, and other people start to practice being content, satisfied, and being grateful.

Chinese parents often teach their children to study hard, and hopefully, later, their child can find a good-paying job, such as lawyer, doctor, IT, financial, etc. In the US, we may see things differently; we encourage children to do what they love to do. Both ways have pros and cons. A high paying job may not be the job the child likes, or the child can handle. For instance (this happened recently), one of my students who used to be a lawyer, quit his job due to heart disease and stroke, then started a business different from the law. Unfortunately, his heart disease was too severe, and several years later, he passed away. Another student went to an Ivy League college, but she could not handle the pressure, and then she quit. One Harvard student (Chinese) killed himself after not being able to handle the cultural differences and his parent's strong feelings. But if children follow the idea "I'll do as I wish," it doesn't matter what the situation, later in life when they grow up, some of them may have a hard time finding a job or career, or may not be able to stay employed, consequently they will be struggling for a lifetime.

I feel that Americans are more realistic, practical; most don't care about showing off. They enjoy who they are, what they do, and don't get bothered by criticism. Now, more and more Americans pay more attention to their health, their wellbeing, and their happiness.

Every child is unique and has their own talent. If we allow for their full skill and expertise, they will do well no matter where they are.

Support system:

For many years, China has had a culture of social involvement. People, friends, and family have always been supportive of each other, helping each other, making suggestions, coaxing you out of a situation if they think it is not a good idea. If you need a job, friends, or family members, try to find connections to get you in. If you don't do well, family and friends try to help you to figure out why you aren't doing well. That can be positive or negative, depending on whether you are following good suggestions or poor suggestions. But at least people try to help.

Regarding looking for a job, generally speaking (in old Chinese tradition) we don't brag about themselves, we try to be modest, show respect, show others we are willing to learn, prepared to work hard. But things have changed, where the old tradition may have lost something. The younger generation is more similar to western culture: they need to tell the world how good they are. In any case, the "people connection" is the same, and it is still essential in looking for a job, starting a new business, or doing business with others. China has changed so much that I don't even know how far China will go.

In the US, things may be different in different states and cities. I heard good things from my students and friends living in different States. I have been living mostly in the Northeast. I have experienced many things in a very different way. People do help each other but to a certain degree. When having a personal or family issue, people tend not to get involved, including relatives. Not many want to share their problems either. From hearing "not my business" so many times, I decided to deal with everything by myself. In some ways, it was good: if I could make it through the toughest things, I could make it through other things. That also made me strong, more independent, and developed strong capability. This also has helped me to be able to help patients who were at a dead end, unable to find their way out. I had many patients who suffer from depression, anxiety, panic. This illness, I did not see so much while I was in China.

Being unable to find answers, many people need to go to "counseling," "therapists" to get answers. I think they may feel better afterward, but they're not getting lasting results in some cases. The good part is that there is much professional help for both physical and mental needs.

When going to a job interview here in the US, we have to elaborate and show everything we are good at; some people even lie to get the job. Otherwise, they may not get hired. But the dishonest person could be eventually fired when the company finds out the truth.

Education and how to present yourself is crucial. Some people take classes on how to interview and get hired; some people take classes to learn other skills if those skills are in high demand in the job market.

Finding Love:

For centuries in China, marriage was arranged. Couples were introduced, usually by parents. Friends, or friends of friends would help to introduce someone who they thought might fit well as a couple. The criteria were: height, looks, how well established, education level, parents' education or financial status, etc. It had little to do with personality. But now things have changed, people have a choice regarding their dating and relationships, including online dating.

The divorce rate was low in the past, whether or not it was a happy marriage or not a happy marriage. Couples often consider their children and don't want to traumatize them. But the divorce rate has increased in the recent 20 years. Compared to the US, however, the divorce rate is still lower.

In the US, there is freedom in choosing a loved one, online dating, bar dating, or meet at a party are all possible. Parents don't get involved too much, but they can share their opinion with their son or daughter regardless of whether the son or daughter will listen or not. Even though there are many happy marriages, the devoice rate in the US is still high. For whatever reason, I believe every failure is a step to success.

I think, and I believe, no matter where you live, love should be based on mutual understanding, mutual respect, and care for each other. It should not be based on money because love is not measured by money. Love is real, is pure, is exceptional energy between the two people that is like magic or a miracle.

Socializing:

Chinese people love to get together, to drink, to eat, to sing Karaoke, or to go places together. They don't drink every day; they only drink during dinner gatherings, often someone gets drunk (called happy drunk: extremely happy, so they have to drink). These kinds of people years later may have liver disease or liver cancer. In recent years people enjoy traveling together more, which is another excellent way to socialize.

In addition to strolling, window shopping, dining together, playing "Mahjong," playing chess, morning exercise, Many Chinese people love to sing; so, Karaoke is very popular in China. Twenty years ago, I was surprised to see so many friends became excellent singers in Karaoke places. People sing to have fun, and that also boosts their adrenaline. They don't worry about how well or how poorly they sing. For a long time living in the US, I did not sing, and nobody sings unless watching professionals and sometimes sing along with them. After seeing most of my friends sang so well, I started to sing (but in Chinese). Singing is a different type of Qi practice, which is very healthy for our body and our mind.

Unfortunately, here in the US, many people are afraid of singing, and their excuse is that they feel they are not good singers and don't want to disturb others. During these years, when I had my clinic and school, I organized many parties throughout the years and included Karaoke singing. Some of my students got over their fear and had a blast singing Karaoke.

Exercise:

For many years in Chinese cities, people always walked or rode bikes from one place to another. Many of them did not feel they needed any extra exercise. Now in China, many people have a car; people who drive have less physical activity, and their health is not as good as people who walk daily. Many Chinese (especially retired people) like to go to the park early in the morning, along with many other people doing all kinds of exercise for about 1 to 2 hours. Looking at these people, you might never guess what age they are. Many of them look ten years younger than their real age.

Now China has gyms in every city; younger people enjoy going to the gym. There are many classes offered everywhere, such as Yoga, Indian dance, ballroom dance, and other kinds of dance exercises.

In America, we are doing better than before. People are starting to pay more attention to their bodies and mind. Gyms are well established, and there are many classes offered there and in other wellness centers. Many martial art studios also offer Tai Chi class, Qi Gong class, and other wellness classes. People do many other outdoor exercises too: hiking, biking, swimming, jogging, walking, boating, and water sports.

Health Care:

Health Care is complicated in both China and the US. China has changed so much regarding health care and health insurance. I didn't hear any complaints from my family about their health insurance in the past ten years nor from my friends. Maybe it is because I did not meet any complainers or people were just too friendly to talk about the negative. Here in the US, I hear so much disappointment with health care and health insurance, including my own experiences. I don't want to criticize but want to share my feeling on how our system is conceived mostly for corporate profit and less for patients benefits. For example, people have to pay out of pocket thousands of dollars on top of paying health insurance premiums. Also, for doctors who are not in the insurance "network," the insurance company will not cover the doctor's visit. Therefore patient, again, will pay out of pocket. That may be ok for people who are financially secure, but not for average Americans. I am sure some insurance is better than others; maybe a university's insurance coverage is better than a private company's. In my own experience, I went to a physical therapist for six visits (prescribed by my doctor after my surgery), then had to submit the bill from the physical therapist who is not in their network. My insurance company rejected the claim saying they require a code and the therapist's professional number. I asked the physical therapist five times: phone call two times, email two times, then letter, to give me the information that the insurance required. However, the physical therapist is just too busy to provide me information but made copies of his notes for each visit. Guess what; the insurance refused to pay. Therefore, I had to pay out of pocket about $1000 for 6 PT visits, even though I have insurance, and the therapy is a prescription by my surgeon. I know I am not the worst case; I heard much worse. Therefore, I am not complaining as long as I am well.

No matter if you have insurance or not, the best way is to stay healthy to avoid complicated battles with the system.

Legal system:

I know that China has improved so much compared with the past. But I have to say America (even though not perfect yet) has a better and complete legal system. China is a big country, and there are many rural communities where there is less formal legal management. Maybe now it is different, but I can't say. Some rural areas in China seem to be lacking. Most cities are well managed, established, and continue to improve, and for this, people are much happier than before. In my experience, I had my wallet stolen by a pickpocket when I was traveling to China, in broad daylight in a public place. Two years ago, my I-phone was taken in Beijing airport while I went through a security check. But I have seen improvement in recent years. I believe China will continue to improve. I have to say in China, no matter where you go or how late you are out at night, it is safe. People, especially younger people, love to go out at night to have a drink, street food, party, watch shows, and they don't need to worry about their safety issue because generally speaking, it is safe at night, in most cities.

In all of the 30 years that I have lived in the US, I have never been robbed. Maybe it's because I don't live in a big city, or perhaps I was lucky, I guess I lived in a safe area. But whatever the reason, I am happy to live where I don't have worry and fear. I cannot say living in the US is safe, especially since many people own guns, and among them, there are some mentally ill people. But you cannot tell who are the mentally ill people. And, if they have not done anything illegal, no one can take their gun away (until they commit a crime). Therefore, it is better not to go out at night or at least have several people together if you do go out. It was so strange in the beginning when I came to the US; I did not see many people out on the street at night, every place was so quiet, and the stores closed early. Then I often thought about China, the night time is the noisiest and you see a lot of people out in public. I assume the farmland is different.

Another thing is, I often hear in the US, people saying "I am tired"; whereas in China, I don't know how people have so much energy, I rarely heard "I am tired." Is this emotional difference or physical difference? I have not figured it out yet. Maybe it is "people."

Environment:

For many years, China had a big pollution problem. The air quality seriously needed to be improved. But in recent years, every year I went to China, I have seen the improvement which made me very happy, to know they are working on this issue. The government moved major manufacturer out of cities, built more roads, more public parks some has outdoor gyms. Unfortunately, more and more people own cars, which leads to continuous pollution. Thinking 1.3 billion people live in China, if everyone has a car, I am not sure there will be any space for parking, driving, repairing, etc.

China is a beautiful country, has many beautiful national parks; some of them are just breathtaking. The only thing is if you visit national parks around holidays, not only is traffic horrific, the national parks are crowded with people, some parks you see more people than scenery. The number of people in the parks certainly creates an issue to keep the park clean. At one time, when I was in a beautiful national park in Hunan province (Zhang Jia Jie, where the Avatar movie has some scenes), I wanted to go home because of the number of people with no space to move around was making me dizzy. I know part of it is my allergy problem, not another problem. But I believe things will change and will be better shortly. China has a terrific leader who knows how to improve things.

In the US, in my experience, every place I go, I enjoy the fresh air, natural habitats, well-maintained parks, abundant greenery. People (majority) have good habits or follow the rules keeping the environment clean. Occasionally, you may see some people do not follow the rules. The national parks are remarkable in the US, it is breathtaking and magnificent, and very clean, well-managed, with easy access and well-thought-out infrastructure. Most public places are clean, convenient, and people are polite, which makes everything more pleasant.

If you use public transportation, people queue up to get on and get off. If someone bumps you by accident, immediately he would say, "I am sorry." Public places, in general, is not loud unless there are children, younger people, or you are at an amusement park. If your car breaks down on the highway, most likely, either a police officer or other drivers will stop to ask you if you need help.

Our homeland (my adopted), where we're raised, we grow up, we work, we retire, and we will be buried. Must be protected. Don't ever let anyone destroy this beautiful land.

Traffic:

In China, even now, with more lanes on the highway, traffic can still be terrible. Around holidays, it is better not to drive in China. On any day, traffic can be bad. It doesn't have to be a holiday. I remember one time my nice Luo Hui kindly drove me to Shu Zhou from Shanghai. Usually, it takes about one hour. But that time, it took us 4 hours back to Shanghai from Shu Zhou. Approaching the toll booth, we sat in the line for 30 minutes waiting for so many cars to pass through., I could not wait any longer to use the bathroom. So, I got out of the car, walking across eight lanes with slow-moving vehicles, and finally found a bathroom at a service area beyond the toll plaza. My niece was scared to death, never seeing anyone do that. But I had to go, even if I had to dodge traffic. I regretted that I complained about the traffic to my niece since she was so kind as to drive me there, and I am sure she was just as frustrated as I was. I forgot to apologize to her too. What a fool I was.

In China, it is better to use public transportation, which is far more advanced and convenient. The Chinese subway system is impressive: safe, comfortable, and inexpensive. Due to the massive population in China, the government builds many tracks for high-speed trains. The high-speed train is fabulous in China; you can easily go almost anywhere you want using a high-speed train. It is undoubtedly a competition with the airline company.

On the highway, I was surprised to see the drivers automatically reduce speed when they see a sign, before, there were very few drivers obey the sign. This is because now there are so many cameras on the highway, and if you violate the traffic law, you have to pay a big fine, or you could lose your driver's license.

In the US, traffic can be terrible in a big city but quite smooth in other places, so I have no complaints. But I have seen so many bad drivers, crazy drivers, so many accidents, especially in Florida. I wish the government would do something or make a law to change this situation.

But public transportation is not as convenient as it could be. The subway system, some cities better than others but in general, is older and breaks down more often. I am not sure if it is a political reason or something else, but we seem to fix things much more slowly here than in China.

Topics of Conversation:

People should be careful about how they talk when traveling to a foreign country. Most casual dialog is similar, but some can offend people. Chinese people tend to talk about everything when getting together with friends. They enjoy a healthy debate without any offensive emotional feelings. They may get a high adrenaline boost from this but rarely do they get angry. They do talk about money and income, and they do like to compare which family has a child went to a famous college or is making more money, and which family has a child making less money. Some of them love to brag about their children or child. They do like to ask personal questions even when they may not know each other that well. I remember many years ago I was on the train in China, a woman kept asking me personal questions, I got annoyed but tried to be polite by giving some answers she wanted, but I had to stop talking. Things like this are less likely to happen with people who are well educated. At that time, I wanted to say, "Mind your own business," but I did not want to upset her, especially since we were both on the train and sharing a berth.

In the US, usually, people don't talk about politics, religion, or money (income). Nor do they talk about something that might stir up an argument. They usually don't get into personal matters unless the other person is willing to share. Common topics may be food, places, weather, nature, museum, art, books, learning subject, scientific news, exciting places to go, and other light topics not getting too deep. But if you have friends who are very close to you and you trust each other, I believe you can talk about anything.

Travel or Sightseeing:

Again, this is not everyone, but my observation because I have traveled with Chinese and Americans.

Chinese people like to see different places both in China and other countries. They enjoy taking photos of famous places in the world or a beautiful place. If you invite them to go again, some would say, "Oh, I have been there; I prefer to go to different places." Some of them have excellent photography skill, almost professional. They enjoy telling others how many places they have visited and show their photos or share photos on social media. I do this too.

When I travel with Americans or Europeans, they like to intensely enjoy the place, "soak in" the natural beauty. They may or may not have excellent photography skills, but they prefer to feel the moment and memorize this moment, stay in the moment, absorb this moment's energy. They may come to the same place, again and again, refreshing their experience. I enjoy this kind of activity and would come to the same places to genuinely enjoy the beauty that mother earth provided to us.

Economy:

I am not an economist, but just from observation, I can see that China now has a strong economy, a healthy workforce, more middle class, and more children going overseas for their education. On the other hand, things are more expensive too; some consumer products are more expensive than in the US.

China has a plan for leading the country to move forward, such as the five-year plan, 10-year plan, 20-year plan. Every time I go back to China, I see changes: more new things, new cars, new technologies, transportation systems, new airports, new roads, new everything. The speed of construction is impressive in the past ten years; things are so much better than before. For example, a bridge in Beijing was worn out but still carrying heavy traffic. The government decides to tear it down and rebuild it. The whole process of building this 1300-ton bridge took them 36 hours. But in Boston, the Longfellow bridge finally was fixed after five years, from 2013 to 2018.

The Chinese government is friendly to other countries and has been making friends with many countries, no matter how big or small. By making friends with these countries, they learn, trade, exchange, and help each other. Before, Chinese people used to talk about not having enough income, but now the average salary (working class) is much improved. Since people have enough money, they travel to all over the world, going to many countries we have not even visited yet. You may see many Chinese when you visit another country. They may be loud, but they are so thrilled. Don't be afraid of telling them, "Be quiet, please," "other people don't like too loud." They will respect your suggestion.

One thing in China that I most enjoy is that I feel safe. I feel no worries and feel relaxed. I know China will continue to grow and improve because they have a plan, they have good leadership, and they have a good team.

China and the US have had a long history of friendship since World War II. There is so much trade between these two countries. There are many Starbucks, KFC, McDonald, Pizza Hut, and more US firms in China; many US-made cars in China, and US students in China. I even sold medical equipment to China a long time ago. There are many consumer products in the US from China too. Some consumer products from China cost less here in the US than in China. That makes things more affordable for US citizens. This is a mutually beneficial relationship that has lasted for many years. We need to cherish this relationship; we should not destroy it.

I am not into politics but have a passion for making our life/health better generation after generation. The US is considered the wealthiest country in the world. We used to be the model for the world, and we were always welcomed by most countries we visited. But recently, that reputation has declined. I could see the difference in people's expressions in the past and recent years when I showed my US passport. I don't have any regret about moving to the US; I am happy to raise my kids here, and I am pleased to live here. But I always feel there is something we could learn from China.

Do we have a plan to make our country improve every year? Do we have a plan to solve problems? Happiness comes from harmony, peace, and united people. Are we united? In this wealthiest country, how many people complain about not having enough money for retirement? To continue to lead the world, we must earn trust and respect from other countries, as we did after World War II. How many allied countries do we have now? How well have we succeeded in making American safe, safe to go shopping, safe to walk on the street? How can we work on creating a harmonious society? How can we teach our children to have more moral behavior, more kindness, and more respect for each other? How can we eliminate drugs? Most of all: how can we strive together as a team?

Overall, both China and the US have strong parts, and both have things that can be improved. If we continue to be friends, learn from each other, helping each other to develop and to grow, we can thrive side by side, to be leading countries and keep the highest reputation in this world.

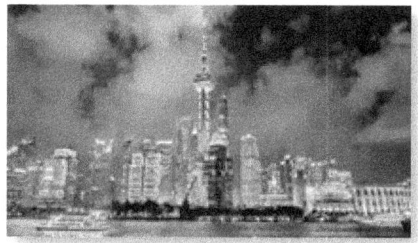 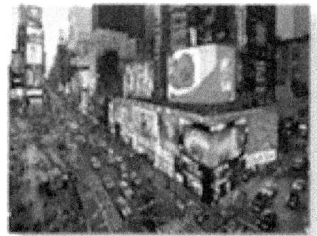

1. Pu Dong, Shanghai
2. Times Square, NY

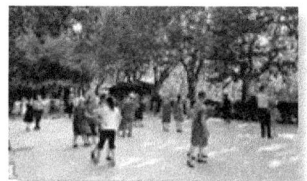 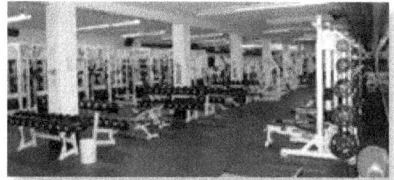

3. Dance Exercise, Hunan, China
4. Weight Training room, USA

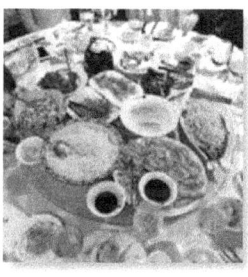 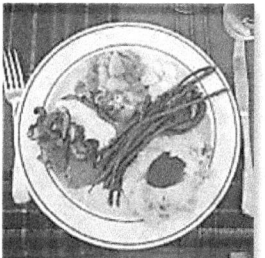

5. Typical Chinese dinner table
6. Typical American dinner

Chapter 17: About My Father

My father was about 5' 7" tall; he was thin. He was a smoker for most of his life, but he did quit in his 50s due to lung disease. He drank about one once of liquor every night, and he loved noodles and dumplings. He loved to drink hot tea, hot soup, and eat spicy foods. I learned in medical school that if you drink liquor or hot liquids consistently, it can burn the esophagus and lead to esophagus cancer. One day I came home and saw my father drinking with his meal. I said to him, half-jokingly, "Do you know that alcohol can cause esophagus cancer." He laughed and said, "I only drink a little." I did not want to take his joy away, and I stopped trying to educate him. Later, he did develop esophagus cancer, and I wished I hadn't said that to him. I felt like I put a spell on him, really regretted it. On the other hand, I knew I could not stop him either.

My father was a special man who will never be forgotten by anyone who knew him. He was always known as a straightforward man, an honest and stubborn man, transparent, with a big heart, and much kindness. Since he participated in World War II fighting the Japanese in China, he attained a high-ranking job. During the cultural revolution, he was accused of being a "capitalist follower," "following capitalist power holders," which I did not understand, because none of the accusations made any sense.

In 1971, he was sent to a "Re-Education Cadre School," also called the "May 7 Cadre School", in a rural area. It was a government-sanctioned program to send cadres to be re-education for their beliefs and ideas through harsh physical labor, mainly farming. My father, along with many other people, did much physical labor. He worked there for one year, feeding pigs, working in the fields, cleaning buildings and office floors, and took mandatory classes daily. Government officials offered the classes;

the intention is to re-mold one's beliefs and ideas. That was like a prison without guards or guns.

During that year, he was away from home, leaving my mother and our siblings. He was down, confused, but sincerely followed the government requirement because he still believed maybe the government is right. He went through ups and downs with transfers from job to job assigned by the government. We had to relocate with him, moving twice in Changsha, then moving to Hong Jiang, then back to Changsha. Regardless of these ups and downs, he still kept his beliefs, which we (my siblings and I) called stupid ideas.

But he was so kind, so patient with us, and always helped us any time we needed it. We loved him and respected him so much. He always asked us how is work, how we felt in life, were there any challenges. If there were any relationship problems between a spouse or siblings, he always asked us to look deep into our self, what did we do wrong to make this conflict or argument; he would ask us to make corrections. If one of us fought with another family, he always took our sibling to the family and apologized to the family; then, he would provide financial re-payment to that family. He never blamed anyone for anything but strictly asked us to improve ourselves.

At work, he put everything into it. Very often, he worked late; even after work, he greeted visitors (workers) to help them solve their problems. He very often offered food for visitors if they came during dinnertime that made my mother upset because she had to make extra dishes for un-expected guests.

He also often helped his relatives in other states. For instance, his brother's grandchild needed a job; he would provide a job in his factory; if they needed money, he would send money. That continued for many years until my mother got angry, she felt there was no end to sending other people money, while he had nothing.

My Father passed away on November 17th, 2000. He died from cancer of the esophagus, colon, then metastasized whole body, he had many other chronic illnesses.

On the evening of November 16th, he was still in the hospital; he was remarkably clear-headed after being sick for so many years. He asked his home care person to bath him and change his clothes; then, he asked her to give him a glass of warm milk even though he could not drink due to the blockage from the esophagus cancer. He forced himself to drink a little. Shortly after, his condition deteriorated. My sisters went to the hospital. He was unconscious. Two hours later, he died at 2:45 AM on November 17, 2000, at the age of 78.

In his will, he wrote, "I don't have too much to request but three things from my friends and family. The first, when I die, don't tell my children who live far away until after everything is settled. The second, donate my body to the medical school for either research or to help students to study Medicine. The third, cover me with the Chinese Communist party flag".

In China, volunteering to donate your body goes against Chinese tradition, and none of my siblings agreed to the donation of his body. He suffered so much, and he gave to his country so much; his whole life was about his country and the communist party, and in the end, the state did not even provide decent medical care. I had to pay much of his medical bill at that time.

He deserved better treatment. But even with his last breath, he was still thinking about how he could help others or benefit others. All my siblings cried and begged him to change his will, but his stubbornness made us speechless, and we did what he wished. He asked to donate his body to the medical school that I attended. When I later saw his will, I cried and cried, I felt worse because my first husband died there; now, here was my father donating his body there. When I found out about his passing, it was two days later when everything was already settled. I did not get the chance to see him. By delaying the announcement, he had spared me the long trip from the US. We visited his grave later.

His funeral was big, with over 300 to 500 people, a lot of flowers, almost everyone cried during his funeral. He had suffered many illnesses for many years, emphysema, COPD, asthma, chronic bronchitis, and bowel disease. He had Tuberculosis when he was nine years old and never had much physical stamina. In 1979 he almost died from pneumonia. About three years before he passed, he was diagnosed with esophageal cancer. He always joked: "I died many times, but God always sends me back" (even though he had no religion). He did not have good physical health throughout his whole life, but he had such a healthy spirit, which is what supported his life year after year. My father was a true believer in Communism. He firmly believed there is nothing wrong with the Communist system. He always taught us, "if there wasn't a communist party, there would be no China, our life wouldn't be as good as it is now." I knew his belief was off the wall, but his faith helped him and supported him.

He told me the story that he was in one of the famous battles fighting with Japanese, later there was a movie about this battle called "Red Sun." He also told me some other stories about how he joined the Chinese army unit called the "New Fourth Army" (Xin si jun) during World War II. I always loved to hear his stories, but I was not always with him; I was either in the countryside, or school, or work, or had my own family. I wish I could have spent more time with him and listened to all of his stories.

He told us to do everything to help our country, our society, and our people, never put ourselves first. He told us to work as hard as we can, sacrifice for the country and communist party, and give our life to the country. In 1995, China suffered a significant economic depression, and people were worried, skeptical about the Communist system. He was the only one (from what I hear) who firmly believed that the economy would get better, Communism will achieve its goal, people's lives will improve. I could see his point; now, the economy is improved. But all of my sisters and brothers and I hated it when he talked about politics, no matter how much he wanted to convince us. We just had to sit there and make-believe we were listening. If we argued, he would argue more. I remembered at one time I was arguing with him that Communism is just good thought, a good dream, but cannot be realistic. He got so angry with me, and seriously gave me a big talk.

His whole life was full of faith, optimism, positive thinking, hard work, strong opinions, goals, and always putting others first. When he was working, I remember he often went to sleep late, not watching TV or doing personal things. He would read or write everything down about his work or plans for work, or someone would drop in to ask him a favor. He had a big job before retiring. Since he was so honest, he sometimes rejected people's requests because the requests were violating the rules. For that reason, some people hated him, or made comments saying that he was stupid, a stone, not flexible. But most people knew he was the most righteous man and admired him. We all knew that China, in the past, had a reputation for "corrupt officials,"; not in my father's case. This man did not fit in a corrupt world; therefore, he was often passed over for promotions.

He criticized me a lot for many things when I was young. He pointed out a lot of my weakness. When I was a teenager, he always criticized me for not reading the newspaper. He criticized me for not being focused, and he would comment if I didn't focus, I could not succeed at anything. He said I wasn't working hard enough; I was too finicky. He said I didn't have modesty; he said that without modesty, I would not learn nor improve myself. He told me every single person has a good part you can learn from, so I shouldn't think how good I am. He felt I needed to build the base of my life, not just floating on the surface. At that time, I did not like it; I hated it. I was just one of the millions of ordinary teenagers. As I grew older and became more mature, I appreciated his teaching/criticizing more, and I realized that he had taught me so much in his own way. Without his criticism and honest opinion, I would not recognize my weakness nor see myself. He was putting a lot of hope and faith in me. I realized the meaning of the name he gave me: "Aihan" (love cold), not to be afraid of challenges. I know that I had the best father, a beautiful gift from God.

In March 1999, my sisters and brothers were notified by the hospital that my father was in critical condition. At that time, he lost consciousness for several days. We were all prepared for the worst. But he surprised us, and he made it through. He was in the hospital for a month. The cost of the stay was above what he could pay. Typically, his health care expenses would have been covered 100% by the company. Unfortunately, the company he worked for was going bankrupt, so they did not pay for his hospital bill. The hospital suggested, "you have a daughter in America, she could pay this for you." My father spoke firmly to them, saying it would be shameful to let an American know this. Even though my father did not ask for anything from me, I knew it was the only way to keep him alive if I sent the money for the hospital bill, as well as supporting his future medical care. So, I did.

He hadn't been eating well for a couple of years due to the blockage of the food passage. In June 2000, I brought my children and my husband to China; that was the last time we all saw him. At that time, he was fragile, and we could see his bones underneath his skin. But even though he was in such bad condition, he kept up a good spirit, a good sense of humor, and tried to have a good conversation with us. All the time during that visit, he did not complain about anything, not at all. But I could see how much he was suffering. My family talked about how unfair it was that the government wouldn't cover the medical bills for my father, who followed the communist path his whole life and gave his life to the party. But my father kept telling us that the Country had problems, but it will be better soon. He asked us not to blame anyone or anything. (Writing this part was not easy, my tears were falling).

His life was frugal and built on faith. He told me he had nothing to leave to us, but two pairs of silver chopsticks. He asked me to teach my husband, and my children learn to use chopsticks to keep in mind Chinese culture and tradition and never forget my Chinese culture and Chinese family. This conversation brought tears to my face, and I did not know what to say. I wanted to say that I don't want anything. I want you to be healthy. But my throat felt like it had a big lump, I could not talk. After I calmed down a little, wiped my tears, blew my nose, allowed my breath to slow down, I asked him if I could have two things from him: the group picture of him and Chairman Mao (the founder and Chairman in China from 1949 to 1976), and his memoir that he would have to write. He was delighted that I asked for these two gifts because no one in my family wanted them.

I only saw him two times in my 14-day family reunion because I could not bear watching him suffer. I cried every time I saw him; it was just too sad; he was too frail. Now I feel so guilty and regretful that I did not spend more time with him. I was too selfish.

I really miss him a lot. I cried every time I thought about him, not because I felt I was one of his favorites, but because I adored him as a good person, full of faith, selflessness, always keeping his inner strength, his kindness, his honesty no matter how much other people said that he was honest to a fault. I respected his loyalty to the Country (China), his love for every family member even though he did not have ways to show it, his belief in China and the system, and his patriotic fervor. Whenever I had a hard time in life, I thought about him. I thought: what would he tell me to do?

My Father: did not leave any money, no possessions. But he left his life story, his spirit, his kindness, and his teaching: belief, keep the faith and work hard!

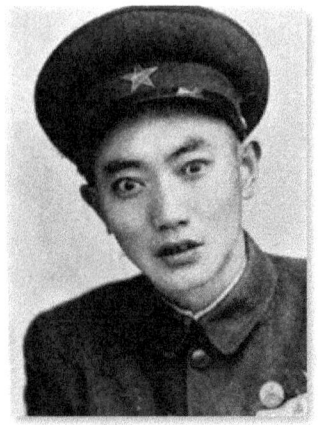 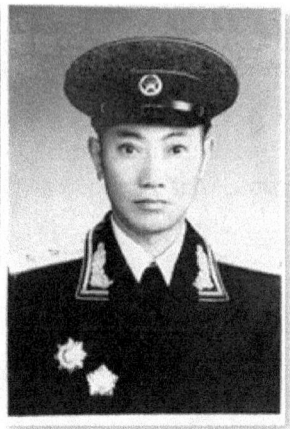

1. Went to the Korean War in 1951
2. Teaching in Military Cadre school 1955 to 1960

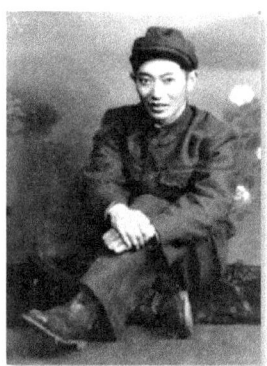 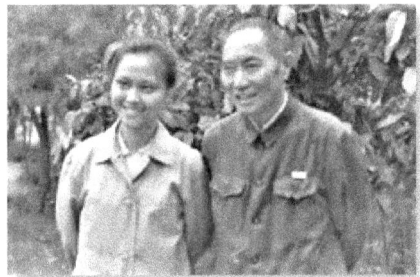

3. My Mom and Aunt took care of sisters during Korea
4. My Dad and me in 1975

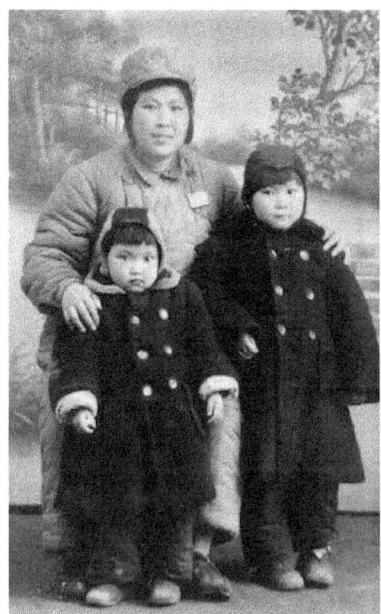

Mother took care of sisters during the Korean War

Chapter 18: My Hip Story

When I was ten years old, I felt my body was very stiff, but I didn't know why. I wished my apartment had a better clean floor so that I could sit there and do some stretching. I envied other kids who were able to do a split because no matter how hard I tried, I could never do a split. I felt my body was made from heavy rubber (like a tire).

I got sick often in my childhood, as well as in my adulthood. Since age 16, I had occasional pain on the left hip, but no doctors (in either China or the US) could find anything wrong. I thought that it was not a big deal. As I got older, the symptoms got worse, but I still did not believe I had a medical issue. I firmly believe I can be better if I continue to do my exercises. Living in the US since 1989, I continued to work, raise children, take care of the family and house; I did whatever women need to do. I noticed my hip pain was getting worse every year. The X-Ray showed I had developed arthritis in both hips, and it is getting worse as the years pass. I thought maybe the cause was the farm work when I was 17 to 21: planting rice in muddy fields with bare feet and without proper nutrition, and also perhaps some genetic deformity.

About the year 1998, one orthopedic doctor told me that it was hip dysplasia; my hip was not well developed. I was born this way. I asked the doctor if there was any cure, but his answer was "No." He gave me some medication for pain. Unfortunately, I had an adverse reaction with severe stomach pain. I could not use the medicine.

In the summer of 2006, while I was still living in MA, I got a tick bite. I pulled the bug off and then used alcohol to wipe the area. I know not everyone will get Lyme's disease, so I believed I might be a lucky one who would not get it. About several months to a year later, I developed severe fatigue, body pain, joint pain. I thought it was cold weather, too many rainy days, or I was working too much.

I love the outdoors, and I love nature. I love plants, flowers, rivers, mountains, and trees. But being outdoors so often, my chance to get Lyme's disease was high. I am the owner of "Chinese Medicine for Health" clinic, and "New England School of Tai Chi" in Massachusetts, and I had to work hard. In 2007, there was one occasion when I had a chance to get a blood test done with a "Darkfield microscope." The test results showed that l had Lyme's disease. I suddenly put together two and two that maybe was why my pain and arthritis were worse. I went to a doctor to ask for a blood test for Lyme's disease, but it was negative. From what I described; the doctor did prescribe antibiotics for ten days. It did nothing for my symptoms. I still had pain, fatigue, and mental exhaustion.

I continued to work, as usual, trying to deny that I had a problem. I was trying to smile, even though I was in pain. It worked! No one (or not many) knew I had any problem. They still loved to hang out with me. At the same time, I decided to help myself by doing more Qi Gong, Tai Chi, targeted stretching, and eating better. It made a difference, and I felt better.

For a long time, I have always paid attention to my health: eating healthy foods, doing exercise regularly, keeping my emotions balanced, and teaching people to do the same thing. This is because I don't have good genes; therefore, I must work hard to manage this and avoid suffering. In addition to my healthy lifestyle, I continuously search for healing methodologies from both eastern and western medicine. I pretty much had tried everything I could to manage my symptoms. I did well most of the time and was able to enjoy my life and work most of the time.

I found a way to deal with my health problems after suffering for so long; I found I can feel better with ancient Chinese therapeutic exercises such as Qi Gong, Tai Chi. I, therefore, became very passionate about these exercises, doing them more often, along with self-healing, self-empowerment, and continuing to grow in my spiritual life. These exercises helped me to reduce my pain too.

I knew I could not be wholly healed with this high-stress job. I made plans to move out of MA and was willing to make some significant changes in my life. When people found out I planned to close my office and was moving to Florida, many people cried, and I cried too. For 17 years, I developed such good relationships and became attached to my students and patients and people working with me. Even now, I still miss these beautiful people up in Massachusetts.

Living in Florida for four years has been very good for me and my health. My symptoms are better; everything is better. Unfortunately, my hips showed in X-Ray severe to near end-stage arthritis. I did not want to believe just one doctor, so I consulted three orthopedic doctors plus other doctors, and all of them suggested surgery. I finally have to accept the fact that I may have to go through surgery, and that was not easy for me to grasp.

On the other hand, I thought about it; this may be a learning experience for me, who never had any surgery before. I decided to proceed with the surgery for one of my hips (the doctor refuse to do both). I scheduled surgery for three months in advance.

Before my surgery, I had to go to a clinic several times, and whenever I went to the orthopedic clinic, I immediately said to myself: I don't belong here. Most of the people there were much older than me. I had to continually tell myself: accept the fact, go with the flow, and everything will be better in the end.

In 2018, I decided to do the surgery. Yes, I was a little scared. I have always been the doctor helping others to feel better, but now I have to be the patient, I am not good at being the patient. After learning what I would have to go through with six months' recovery time, not doing most things I usually do for at least three months, needing to take pain killer for a while, my spirit was very low. I felt sad, down, could not sleep. I had so much to do, to write, to teach, and my hobbies: my garden, enjoying nature…

Two weeks before surgery, I was anxious, nervous, and fearful. I never had any surgery, I even helped patients avoid surgery, then helped them to heal, and I always kept things holistic. Parts of my anxieties were from worry about the anesthesia, not knowing what to expect after surgery: would I be worse or better, and what if something happened during surgery. I have a mild form of COPD, asthma, many allergies: dog, cat, mold, dust, and some foods. The general anesthesia involves inserting a small tube into the trachea, and my trachea is very sensitive. I was worried about my breathing during anesthesia. This was one of the most fragile periods of my life in the US. I have always been active and capable, and always able to help others to be better, but I was feeling a loss of my strength. This whole emotional imbalance was very difficult. I always teach people to keep their emotions balanced because emotional health affects physical health and healing. I felt terrible, not being able to adjust myself. I kept reminding myself again and again: be strong, be tough, everything will end well, and my health will be restored.

To ease my anxiety, I bought some blooming orchids (even though I have so many of them), I spent a lot of time taking care of my garden because I knew I wouldn't be able to do much for a while after the operation. The most anxious time was three days before. After talking to my former classmate (who is an anesthesiologist, Dr. Gu, who is currently working in Boston Medical Center), I felt better. My local students were so supportive and kind, and they gave me strength too. I am very grateful.

On the day of surgery, which was Monday, November 26, 2018, I got up at 4:00 AM and took a shower with antibiotic soap as directed, and my husband drove me to the hospital. The registration and pre-surgical work took two hours. The surgery took about 1.5 hour. It was smooth, and I had a new left hip: both hip socket and femur head were replaced with titanium and porcelain.

I returned to my room and woke up by 11:00 AM, but I had no feeling in my leg. That was good, no pain! I was able to smile and talk. In the afternoon, a Physical therapist came to room asked me to do a little walk, telling me to walk a few steps to get the blood moving, I started to feel some pain after walking. That evening was not pleasant: all the anesthetic effect was gone, and I had much more pain, even with pain medication. After taking stronger pain medication that contained an opioid, I fell asleep. I know an opioid is not a good drug and is highly addictive, but I had no choice: I needed to sleep! The doctor prescribed this kind of pain killer for most surgical patients.

On day two, which was Tuesday, a nurse gave me some medication. I was so drugged I didn't even bother to ask what the medicine was. I knew there were pain killers among them. My leg muscles were severely bruised, just like if you got hit by a car; my nerves had trauma, and part of my bone was removed. The pain was inevitable. The staff were very courteous and professional. One nurse's aide was extremely friendly, kind, and caring. The hardest part was getting up and down for trips to the bathroom. Luckily, I did not have any complications. The day was okay, but the evening was worse. I tried not to use too much pain killer by not showing my pain, but by 10:00 PM, the pain brought out my tears, I cried. The nurse gave me a pain killer with an opioid; I then was able to fall asleep. From suffering this pain, I feel like I understand why there is a drug addiction problem nationwide. I decided to defeat this, and I wanted to prove that anyone can avoid addiction. So, I decided to take the minimum of medication. If the pain comes, I tried to breathe, do some Qi Gong on the bed, or try to sleep.

I had the worst food ever in the hospital: green banana, chicken with no flavor, vegetable from a frozen package, or not fresh. I thought a hospital might have a nutrition program for patients, but I was wrong. I ended up eating most of the food that I had cooked previously and asked my husband to bring it for me.

On Wednesday (day three after surgery), I got out of the hospital and went home. The next day I had a home visiting nurse and PT.

At home, I tried only to use Tylenol to manage my pain unless I couldn't sleep at night; this is when I needed one medicine with the opioid. I then tried to skip a day to avoid using opioids every day. I thought if I don't sleep one day due to pain, I will use the opioid the next day. It seemed like a good plan.

By Friday, I felt a little stronger, and the pain was a little less. I decided to do Qi Gong to strengthen my body and raise my energy level. I felt stronger both in my body and my leg muscle with the Qi Gong and the exercise that the physical therapist taught me. I started to take Chinese herbs for my Liver, Kidney, and Spleen (TCM). The prescription medications I was taking can harm the Liver, Kidney, and Spleen. I wanted to protect my organs and my immune function.

There were six physical therapy home visits within two weeks after my surgery; the first four visits were to move my leg muscles when lying down: toe up and down, press heel, press knee down, squeeze gluteus muscle. The last two visits were sitting and standing work: lifting leg, stretching leg.

Things continued to improve, and each day I was getting a little better and stronger.

On day 8, I started to do Tai Chi Walk, horse stance, and try to do a little Xinyi stance. At home between PT visit, I needed to continue my Tai Chi walk and Qi Gong. There are four types of Tai Chi Walk, and I was able to do tai chi walk I (forward) and III (backward) with the help of a walker. Tai Chi Walk is terrific, and I built up the strength of my Quadriceps without pain. I knew there would be some pain if I did too much. Therefore, I limited my walking to doing a little bit between hours. I was so excited with Tai Chi walk; it gave me confidence, strength, reduced pain, and helped me to heal faster. I no longer had any negative feelings about my healing, and I stopped using the pain killers on day 10. I tried to cook meals with the help of my husband. I would do whatever I could and decided to go out and get some sun whenever I could. I tied to do some writing if my pain was not bad, and my mind was clear. I tried to practice piano 10 to 20 minutes each day, even though I am just a beginner.

Nighttime was the worst. The pain was always the worst at night due to the lack of distractions. Sometimes I cried from frustration and then told myself: tomorrow will be better, just hang in there. Every night I say same thing to myself: tomorrow is better, just hang in there. It worked because I convinced myself it would be better.

During my healing, I had great support from friends, family in China, my local students, my distant students, and my husband. That helped me a lot.

On day 10, I tried to walk alternately with and without the walker. But I had to hold onto the wall, counter, chair, or anything that could support my balance. When I had pain, I lost my balance.

On day 11, I tried to use crutches, that gave me a little more freedom of movement.

After 14 days, I was able to put on long pants by myself; after 21 days, I was able to put on socks by myself. I changed from crutches to a cane and had more freedom.

I started to drive to my first outpatient physical therapy on day 18. I had some relief from pain after three weeks of physical therapy (6 visits), which gave me the confidence of healing.

Not being able to do much except cook with the help of my husband, I watched many TV series. I don't regularly watch TV series; usually, I have no time. But the surgery gave me time to enjoy some TV series.

Christmas Eve was four weeks after my surgery. I had a wonderful time at my house with some friends. Even though I had more pain from some cooking, but it was worth the enjoyment.

On day 31, I started to walk without the help of the cane. Not perfect walking, but it gave me more confidence.

I continued to do Qi Gong, Tai Chi Walk, stretching daily, and going to the PT 1 or 2 times a week. My healing was well on the way.

One experience I had during this process was astonishing: the doctor who performed surgery on my hip did not visit me after surgery. Instead, he sent a physician's assistant to visit me and take notes. I had so many questions about my surgery but could not get answers. That made me stressed, uncomfortable, anxious, and those negative emotions affected my healing. Later I decided to write to him and ask those questions in my letter. In my letter, I also expressed my disappointment. After mailing the letter, I decided to let go of my negative emotions, refocus on my healing, do exercise every day, and try to get well. It was amazing to see the difference after having removed my negative emotion and refocus: I felt much better!

During this whole process, I got much support from my husband, who helped with me whatever I needed, my friends/students brought flowers, foods, many emails filled with good wishes. All these made me feel loved. I am grateful for having wonderful friends, students, and my family.

Through this experience, I could see the importance of both eastern and western medicine. To obtain better care and a better quality of life, integrating both medicines makes a big difference in recovering and healing. I also understand now how expensive it is to go through surgery, how frustrating to deal with insurance, why so many people are unhappy with health insurance, why so many of them carry the fear of not being able to pay for insurance or cannot retire earlier because of the insurance worries. Luckily, I had medical insurance but still had to spend a considerable amount.

For me, going through this surgery was part of my learning and experience. Even though I still have discomfort after surgery, I am happy to be able to heal positively. I proved the Daoist way: no matter how hard it is, there will be an end to the hardship.

Part IV Tips for Happiness and Success

Chapter 19: What Brings True Happiness?

If you ask someone, "Are you happy"? Most likely, the person will reply, "yes." We are very private, very secretive, don't always want other people to know our whole life story or our private life. True happiness is not just saying "I am happy"; it is instead living with enduring contentment; it's an inward practice of lifelong satisfaction and happiness.

For centuries, we (most people) were always thinking that money is the way to bring happiness. Therefore, we worked tirelessly to provide abundance to our family. We automatically assume our family should be happy with what we have done for them or provided for them. When we realize things are not like what we expected, we feel deprived, depleted, puzzled, then depressed. We then ask our self: is there such a thing as "True Happiness?"

True happiness is not about having more money, owning more properties, having more possessions, or being a star. Money does support human living, and it can provide us with a comfortable life, allow us to do things we want to do, and help us to buy material things. But money cannot buy happiness. It may buy temporary happiness, which does not last. We do need money to pay bills, make a living, and make sure we have enough when we retire.

But in some cases, money can destroy lives too. Having material possessions is not always the more, the merrier. For some people it is the opposite: the more we have, the more stress we have. Being a star, you get fame and fortune, but your stardom and money can only give you temporary happiness, and shortly after that, it disappears if you don't know how to find true happiness.

Material life is superficial; a spiritual experience with ethical living standards is rooted, of high value, and is in a higher realm. Some people destroy others to climb higher; some kill animals then sell the parts to make vast sums of money. Some steal other's valuables and goods. And some hike up prices for huge profits because they can, while others have to pay due to critical health issues. These people get their money, but they have the least worth to me because they don't have any ethical standards.

To obtain true happiness, we need to understand some fundamentals and work at it.

We need to have good health, both physical and mental.

Good health means everything. Good health includes both physical and emotional aspects. How do we achieve that? Just ask yourself: Do I exercise regularly? Do I have too much stress? How is my emotion? Do I eat well, eat healthy? Do I have negative thoughts periodically? When you have these answers, you can make needed changes. If the answer is contrary to finding happiness, you may be able to make some decisions that lead to happiness. Exercise regularly, whether it is western or eastern forms of exercise, you will feel the difference in your emotion and energy. You can choose to do whatever activity you like: jogging, walking, running, swimming, tennis, ball game, hiking, Tai Chi, Qi Gong, martial art, aerobics, yoga, stretching, even dancing. The key is: you need to do it, and do it regularly.

We need to have good friends.

We all have some friends throughout our lifetime; when we have like-minded friends, our happiness index increases. When like-minded people get together, energy sparks and the health benefit abound. But, be careful, if you are with people who have the same interests but are not living a healthy life, you may feel happy at the time, but you may eventually lose out. I am referring to those who are suffering from alcohol abuse or drug abuse. To find true happiness, the people you chose to stay with should also be health conscious.

Over time, some friends leave, and some friends stay, and some new friends come into your life. This is a normal process. If you and your friends have different energy and a different mindset, or you don't have a similar philosophy of life, either you or your friends may leave the relationship. This is a normal process and part of life. There is no need to be upset or angry. The disappointment and anger can only hurt you and make you unhappy. The wisdom here is: the more you force things, the less you get. Just let your body and mind rest for a while; go with the natural flow, and your happiness will be eventually be restored. Some friends can be forever friends who you always enjoy talking with and seeing. This is the lucky part of your life, cherish it. Some new friends come into your life, you feel good about making new friends who may be perfect or not exactly right. It takes time to know and understand a person. The bottom line is kindness. Without this, a friendship cannot last.

When making friends, you should never think, "How is this useful for me"? Make friends with your heart, and you will have good friends. If you make friends by analysis, you may not have any real friends. With true friends, you can share stories, have heart to heart conversations, spend time together, and be there for each other. Genuine friendship is giving, not just taking. Real friends help each other go through hard times, encourage each other to move forward, and are not afraid to tell a friend what needs to be improved. Real friends may not always praise you. But they do tell you the truth even when you may not want to hear it; because they want to help you in your growth and achievement. When you have true friends, you don't have to play mind games with each other, and you can be as honest as a little child. That is true friendship, and true friendship lasts forever.

Positive friends give you energy; negative friends reduce your energy or deplete your energy. Having the mindset of "using each other," is not true friendship; it is a business relationship which is a superficial level of friendship.

We need to have a positive attitude.

Have you heard of the expression: "Attitude is everything?" I've heard it many times, and I teach it many times too. Everything has two sides: good or not good (or bad), but there is no absolute good or bad. Most of the time we spend in our lives, hopefully, is to create good things, but we go through bad things too, this is a life journey. On our journey, we may have an easy path, or we may have a difficult path. We may meet wonderful people, and we may meet a few terrible people. We may do something just right, and we may make mistakes. But no matter what we go through, the journey always seems to become easier each year or each decade. Even when you feel the worst at one moment, you know the worst will pass; or if you reach a high point, you know you may drop. Just be calm, be present, and be part of the natural process of ups and downs, you will be able to maintain a balanced energy level. There is no need to over-analyze everything. Instead, be observant, let the natural process take you to wherever it is going.

It is easy for other people to say "don't be negative, be positive," but it is a journey and a mindful practice to be positive. No one is perfect, we all have some good days and bad days, and we all try to find a way to deal with the bad days. We sometimes overcome the bad days; other times, we may feel stuck. In my experience, I did Qi Gong or Tai Chi when I felt stuck or had a bad day. I felt much better after my Qi Gong and Tai Chi practice. That was why I wrote the book "Tai Chi for Depression," which is available on Amazon and in bookstores. I also always keep in mind the Daoist teaching, "Everything will pass."

On our journey, we continue to learn, to grow, to make changes, to figure it out and learn, and to find our perfect world inside of us: true happiness. You will finally realize: yes, it is true that attitude is crucial.

We need to have love.

Love goes both ways: we receive love, and we give love. To receive love, we must know how to love others. To achieve this, we must know how to give, to forgive, and to be honest with ourselves and others; this way, you earn trust and love. Love also involves understanding, nurturing, and selflessness.

Over the years, I have seen many cases where people who tend to give are happier than people who tend to take. Easy-going people are healthier than those who are tense or stressed. When you help other people or give to people, you automatically create positive energy. The positive energy makes you feel good and happy. If you think you lose something by helping others, or if you are worried that you are giving out too much and not getting back, or if you try to calculate if it is fair or not fair, you create tension and stress that causes blockages in your body, in your mind, in your life, in your relations and your health. Calculating "how much do I get?" weakens your spirit. Life is not just "another day, another dollar." Giving is priceless, it is from your heart, and nothing can measure the value of giving. You are happier when you have something to offer.

Giving and forgiving go together. If you only give but not forgive, you only practice 50%, and that doesn't get you to genuine love. "True forgiveness includes total acceptance. And out of acceptance, wounds are healed, and happiness is possible again." --- Catherine Marshall (author). Forgiving others creates positive energy, and it is the practice of letting go, which provides you with health benefits. We all make mistakes in our lives, and we all learn from our mistakes. Love increases when you practice forgiveness, and forgiveness nurtures love.

When you hold onto negative thoughts from the past, you create blockages in your mind like a bird locked in a cage with no freedom. The blockages in mind eventually harm the body causing physical illness. Once you can forgive and let go, you set yourself free; your mind is open and free, and your energy channels are opened, and your happiness and love can be restored.

Truthfulness with yourself and with others is another essential practice to set free your mind; this also earns people's trust. No one likes to be with someone who wants to play mind games, deceiving, and boasting. Truthfulness and honesty can set you free from chaos and make life easier.

"Love comes when we take the time to understand and care for another person."
—Janette Oke (a Canadian Author of inspirational fiction).

Love involves understanding, nurturing, supporting, giving, and caring. Without any doubt, practicing these can not only create a long-lasting love but also create a supportive environment for health and healing. No matter how long or how short your marriage is, you should always respect each other, cherish love, give in and make necessary concessions because you need each other, and you never know when you may lose one another in this chaotic world. With love, compassion, conscientiousness, and moral strength, any relationship can endure.

There are different kinds of love, beyond just couples. There is love between mother and daughter or son, love between husband and wife, love between friends, love between siblings, and love between you and your pet. All these kinds of love can be appreciated and cherished. Giving love is the basis for receiving love.

If you are looking for a lifetime companion, you should look for someone who understands love, knows how to love, is kind, sincere, deep, and has a high standard of self. Not just for the sake of getting married to someone similar. If you're looking for a "money man," your happiness may be temporary. Love is not measured by how much money there is; it is measured by two hearts being in sync, in harmony, and unity. Nothing can break apart two beautiful hearts if you find the right one. Someone who loves money more than you, cannot bring true love; it is not worth it to go through the trouble unless you want to. Temporary pleasure does not last. Once you have sincere love, both of you can work, can make money, can build a beautiful home and life. For women, my opinion is, your guy should be gentle, kind, caring, understanding, sincere, have a good heart, a good work ethic, and be able to communicate in a healthy way. It is not a good idea to have someone in your life with a bad temper, alcoholic, drug user, ego-centric, manic, or womanizer. Either male or female, if you value life and love, you will find ways to make things better. Anyone can have choices in his/her love life. If you still do well after 30 years of marriage, you must have done something right. If you fail, it would be a lesson for you, but sometimes a harsh lesson.

Love is precious, pure, and unconditional. It is the highest power that can bring two people together on their journey, and it helps us to overcome all obstacles on this journey. It should always be protected.

We need simplicity, harmony, balanced emotions, and inner peace.

Yes, we do need simplicity! Life becomes more complicated every year; not only is there too much happening in our life but also, we create complications for ourselves by overloading our mind by overthinking and over-analyzing. Furthermore, we weigh ourselves down with activities to the point where we realize we can't breathe. Our emotions go up and down and sometimes become chaotic or imbalanced.

There is a significant difference between western psychology and Daoist psychological healing. Western psychology tries to analyze everything, looking for reasons for everything. Sometimes, when you work so hard to find a reason or try to find the exact answer, try to be so smart, you create an ongoing battle within yourself. You may understand the cause of the problems but may not know how to get past them. Things happen for reasons and can be solved with smart living: Daoist healing wisdom.

Some people worry about things that may never happen, which is a complete waste of energy. Cautiousness is a good habit to have to deal with unexpected situations, but being overcautious creates tension in your mind, which eventually creates blockages in the body energy pathways and consequently may cause illness. Our brain is already too busy with so much going on in life, but if we continue to overthink, worry too much, plan too much, and fear too much, our thought process may become inefficient, even trigger depression, anxiety, or panic attacks.

Emotions affect everything, including relationships, as we all may have experienced: ups and downs and emotional waves created in a relationship. Emotion can also affect career, affect decision making, and affect health. If you realize that you have more emotional ups and downs than usual, it is best to consult doctor or other help. My program, "Emotion Healing," had changed many people's lives, and energy, and you may like to look into it. Keep in mind, nothing is permanent, and things will change, everything changes. Just for this reason, you should not be so hard on yourself. For some people, if you think that alcohol and drug can make you happy, you are very wrong because it is the opposite: making you feel worse afterward, and it can destroy your life, marriage, and career. And, you may never be truly content as long as you drink or use drugs. That is the truth.

We cannot control everything that happens or happened in the past, cannot predict everything that may occur in the future, but we can be prepared with our knowledge. Some people over analyze everything which, to me, is wasting energy. It's better to preserve our energy for important things, such as things we need to do, need to fix, need to prepare, and things we want to do, things for our health, happiness, and well-being. When something happens, we will find ways to deal with it.

Stress is the number one cause for developing an illness. Chronic stress can cause cancer; this has been studied and confirmed by scientists. We have a choice to create a less stressful life, and I have seen people do just that by simplifying their life and mind. Stress comes from our response and our reaction to what is happening. If we don't react or don't respond so fast, both externally and internally, we may be able to figure out how to reduce our stress. Even though the external stimulant is there, it does not affect our life. We do what we have to do. In the past, I reacted, yes, I did have stress and stress did affect my body and emotion. Later, I made changes; my stress is less every year.

Do you feel our free time is less and less? I do. We have too much going on, especially in our internet world. New apps, new distractions, nonstop social media, dealing with hackers and malware, computer or software update/upgrade, etc. There is too much stuff we have to take care of, to deal with, and to fix. Therefore, we have less time to enjoy our life, to read, to exercise, to cook healthy meals, and to socialize physically. These things certainly bring more stress to our life. But we can manage it by being smart.

How to simplify our life?

It has to start with our minds. The mind needs to relax, needs to rest, needs to be quiet, needs to be balanced, and needs to think less. Once the mind is at peace, you feel happy, and you don't feel you need more. If your mind is too busy, nothing can make you satisfied, no matter how much you have. A relaxed mind helps in making the right decisions; the right decisions help you to identify what you need and what you don't need. When you know what you don't need, you can easily simplify your life.

Anthony Bourdain, a TV journalist, specialized in food worldwide. We all thought he had the best job: eating good food every day, traveling the world, and meeting all kinds of people. But he was not able to shake off his stress and did not focus on healing his depression.

Comedian Gilda Radner was so funny and so famous in her career years. I liked her a lot because she had such a natural humorous personality. Her life and health were up and down but never easy. Sadly, she died from cancer in 1989 at age 42. Before she passed, she realized that her mind and emotion were too complicated.

To practice simplicity, one must start by simplifying their mind, then avoid excesses, avoid complications. When you reach that point, you feel lighter, happier, and have more time for enjoyment. Everything should be done in moderation; excess can cause trouble, including over-partying: over-drinking, over-eating, then in time, your health begins to decline.

"Inner peace is the key: if you have inner peace, external problems do not affect your deep sense of peace and tranquility. Without this inner peace, no matter how comfortable your life is materially, you may still be worried, disturbed, or unhappy because of circumstances".

------- *Dalai Lama*

We need to bring more humor into our life.

We are too solemn, too uptight, too restricted, and we overthink. I was like this before, but I am much better now after learning. In the past years, I had many patients come in for a consultation, and I saw some patients were so nervous, anxious, and could not relax. I needed to make them relax so that they could explain things to me clearly. So, I learned to crack some jokes, and made some fun of myself, and talked to them with some humor. It worked! After some laughter, they were more open, more relaxed, and able to tell me their stories in a coherent way. In 2015, I wanted to learn more about speaking with humor and making people laugh, so I decided to take some classes at the local Comedy Club. I took a 9-hour "Comedy Boot Camp "over several weeks. It was presented to learn how to tell jokes lasting 4 to 5 minutes. All 15 students were Americans, and I was the only Asian. Students needed to go on stage one by one and tell a joke for 4 minutes. The goal was to make everyone laugh. All (but not me) told dirty jokes some of the jokes I could not even bear to hear because we (Chinese people) don't say nasty things in public. But the thing is everyone laughed at these off-color jokes, and no one was offended. My jokes were the cleanest, but not many laughed. At that time, I could not overcome my "doctor's manner." Then I thought, what would I lose if I tell some dirty jokes? To come to this comedy boot camp is to learn how to be funny, not to show "doctor's manner."

On the last day, when all of us had to perform at the club that night, I spent the whole day changing my joke by adding some mid-level dirty words and raunchy stories. I also invited some of my friends and my students to come see me at that evening's "Student comedy Show." Guess what, people laughed watching my comedy performance! Yea! All my students said I was great, but my husband emails back to me after watching the clip I sent to him, "Honey, you are not supposed to say those things." I had to email back, "Honey, that is a comedy show, not a speech."

There is no need to be too serious about everything. The only things we need to be serious about is our continuous improvement, working professionally, learning always, and treating each other with sincerity and respect.

We need to set ourselves free.

Living in a country that so values "Freedom," we should feel free. But many of us don't feel "free," because we are influenced in so many ways. When I say we don't feel free, I suppose it's because many things control us. The commercial world controls us with endless advertising. Health insurance companies tell us which doctor to see to be covered for a portion of the bill. Pharmaceutical companies dictate the price of the medicines we need. The government regulates many aspects of our lives. We depend on the food industry, and we believe all foods in the market are safe. We are subject to our own fear, anger, anxiety, worries; we are controlled by our own emotions or negative mindset that can create hate, anger, and illness. If we continue to be controlled by either external or internal forces, we put ourselves in a box that we cannot escape.

How do we get out of the box?

You need to start with your mind. Identifying what controls you is the first step, and after that, it is you who decides if you want to continue to be restrained or you don't want to be controlled. For instance, when someone tells you that you should not do something because you don't have the skill or talent. You may say, "You're, right, I am not good at this," you have then admitted that you are willing to be limited. What if you want to do this work and are ready to put effort into doing it, you may surprise people. I never intended to write a book or give speeches because I was not very good at either written or spoken English. But I am doing it, and I even got awards.

Do you want to buy a second house for investment because your friends bought one and they made money? Must you do what your friends do, or do you wish to be simple and have time and money for other things you like to do? Is it stressful, or not a problem?

Sometimes you may be controlled by old unwanted memories, previous trauma, failure, or unfortunate events. But if it is past, why should you continue to play these old tapes? Letting go can be difficult, but it is possible and definitely will restore your happiness. Being able to let go of the past is the first step in moving forward.

We sometimes are controlled by our expectations, but reality does not always match expectations. It is more satisfying to lower your expectations.

In medical care, you know the medication's side effect will affect you, but your doctor may insist that you take it, what should you do? I know what I would do, but I'm not sure about you.

Think about peer pressure, are you willing to be controlled by the crowd, or do you want to be yourself and not to be swayed by others? It is your choice to be restrained or to set yourself free.

Being controlled may make you happy for a short time, but when you set yourself free, your happiness will last long term,

Here is a Daoist story I heard a long time ago:

A King had a dream. In his dream, an immortal wise man told the King one sentence and asked the King always to remember this sentence because it leads to lifelong happiness. After a night's sleep, the King forgot the sentence. He then told all the palace officials, "if anyone can find this sentence, I will give you a big diamond ring worth $1000.00". One day a wise official came to the King and said: "Give me the diamond ring, I found your sentence." He took the diamond ring and carved the words inside the diamond ring. Afterward, he gave the ring back to the King and left. The King looked at the writing engraved on the ring, and he realized this is what he forgot in his dream: "Everything will pass." (Your glory will pass, your suffering will pass, your difficulty will pass, your humility will pass. We should enjoy the present, embrace life now, cherish what we have now).

We need to set high moral standards for ourselves.

What does this mean? Living with concern for the principles of right and wrong behavior; and the goodness or badness of human character, your "happiness index" is always going to remain at a high level.

Most of us live our lives with moral standards, but in some populations, we have seen unimaginable human behavior. Some people may try to explain it, saying some people have mental problems, but why do we have so many who are mentally ill? How do they develop issues so severe to the point of killing others?

To make life less stressful and more enjoyable, as political leaders or the general population, we need to think about how we can live with honorable, righteous, principled, honest, respectful, truthful, ethical, pure, blameless, and moral behavior.

There was a saying, "He who has no morals cannot be trusted."

I remember during my childhood, both at school and home, I was taught how to be an honest person, be kind to people, and do the right thing.

"Kindness is a passport that opens doors and fashions friends. It softens hearts and molds relationships that can last lifetimes". .... *By Joseph B. Wirthlin*

"One of the toughest things for leaders to master is Kindness. Kindness shares credit and offers enthusiastic praise for other's work. It's a balancing act between being genuinely kind and not looking weak". .... *By Travis Bradberry*

"The beauty of a woman is not in a facial mode, but the true beauty in a woman is reflected in her soul. It is the caring that she lovingly gives the passion that she shows. The beauty of a woman grows with the passing years". ………….. *By Audrey Hepburn*

With moral practice, you become a good person, a trustworthy companion, a likable person, an honorable leader, and a great role model; you will have genuine friends and enjoy a happy life. (People will remember you forever).

We need more nurturing, not fighting.

We have been fighting too much: World War I, II, Korean War, Vietnam war, Afghanistan war, Iraq war; now we have "Trade War." What will be the next war? There are many kinds of fighting of different types and in different places, between different groups, and even in schools (kids fighting). We often use the word "fighting" in the medical field too: fighting cancer, fighting arthritis, fighting heart disease. Let's think for a moment; can we fight when we don't feel well? How about we change the word from "fighting" to "healing"? Can you feel the energy shift?

When you have a "fighting" mind, your happiness index decreases, partially from the tension in your mind and body; when you have a "healing, nurturing" mentality, your body relaxes automatically, and the consequence is you feel happier. Relaxation leads to healing.

Verbal fighting, email fighting, social media fighting are different kinds of fighting, and they also hurt others. Why do we need to hurt others? What benefit do we get from hurting each other or fighting with each other? How about we do things differently? Using words to hurt others shows you are the one who does not have good manners; it also shows you have a negative mindset. But the good thing is that you can change, and you can make things better. You can start with one step at a time; then, you change the energy in you and the people around you.

Why do so many of us have anger or hate? Does anger/hate help anything? Keep in mind that every time you lose your temper, you throw away your happiness. Hate creates so much negative energy; not only does it make you seem unkind to those around you, but you may also develop a disease. Also, life can be tough for those who often have anger or temper tantrums.

The thing that is not appropriate is that you are putting your frustrations towards another person/people. This happens quite often in both men and women. (I did this before, but I realized that it was wrong, I then made changes). Your frustration comes from the fact that you are unable to figure out how to solve your problems, and it has nothing to do with other people. When you do this, your moral image is diminished.

We need more love, nurturing, and healing so that we can restore our happiness, have better emotions, and have a more productive life.

We need to keep our inner child alive.

No matter how old or how young we are, there is no need to say, "I am too old for that." We don't need to admit that we cannot do certain things like younger people. We can do many more things others can't. We can still happily keep our mental sharpness, strength, and wisdom for happy living. Even though it is a reality that everyone will get old eventually, older people do amazing things, and some do what children do too. I remember I once told my friends that I went to Disney World and loved it. My Chinese friends said to me, "Oh, that is kid stuff." With that fixed mindset, they don't get to have fun like children, and they lose their opportunity to experience the exciting moments like young people or kids. I not only had fun but also tested myself to see if my energy is still there like young people: how far and how fast could I walk like more youthful people. Not in a competitive way, I just wanted to see.

We should continue our learning in art, music, singing, dancing, language, reading, doing projects, traveling, hiking, sightseeing, gathering (not drinking gathering), but we don't need to look at our phone 24/7 like young people. At least we can do more thinking and preserve our vision and gain more time, that is what I think.

If you feel happy and satisfied with your life, comfortable with who you are, don't have too many desires, and are not resentful, you must have done something right to get there. But if you have goals and want to achieve your goals, want to continue to improve yourself, the next chapter, "Golden Tips…." may be helpful.

Money cannot buy happiness; money can only provide you with temporary satisfaction. True happiness comes from within you, your internal practice, your effort, your wisdom, and your kindness.

You do need a career, purpose, or goal. You do need to stabilize your economic and financial position for living, which helps you to minimize your stress paying bills. You need to do well with your career, job, and goals. I hope the next chapter may help you.

Chapter 20: Valuable Tips for Success in Life and Career

For many years my idea of success was: go to school and get a degree, then find a job, pay bills, have a family, try to make more money to pay more bills, try to buy property, make our house look as good as the neighbors' house, and that will be "Success." But how many people are truly happy following this old model? It took me many years to figure out that the old way of living is not the way to achieve "Success." Why do I say that? It is because after seeing so many different kinds of patients and getting to know them, I could see many of them had money but suffered from depression, anxiety, and poor health. I finally concluded that real success does not come just from money; it is much more involved. What I believe now by saying "Reach for True Success" is: go to school, learn all kinds of skills, improve your ability to do things, take on challenges both in life and in career, love what you do (do what you love), do it well, improve your abilities in other areas including problem-solving skills, and work for enjoyment.

I once had a patient who had an excellent job in Boston, where I had an office downtown. At one of his appointments with me, he asked me a question. I had answered pretty much every kind of question before, but this time I was stuck, I could not believe it. His name was Tim. Tim said to me, "Dr. Kuhn, Can I ask you a question"? I said, "Sure," with my usual confidence. Tim said, "Why do we live"? My brain was suddenly frozen; I did not know how to answer his question at that moment. Since I did not want to disappoint him, I came up with an answer, but it was not the answer I wanted to give him. I said, "Well, God made us, God wants us to live, so we live." He was not convinced, but he did not say anything either. It was the most awkward moment I had since coming to America because I was stuck, and I did have the answer the patient needed. After that, I thought about it over and over. Finally, I came to a conclusion, at least I think it is the right answer (to me it seems right):

Life is about all kinds of experiences: hard or soft, bitter or sweet, difficult and easy, happy times and troubled times, success and failure; it is like food with all kinds of flavors sweet, sour, hot, bitter, salty, etc. From these experiences we learn, we grow, we become strong, capable, and competent.

I wish I could go back to that time at my Boston office to give Tim that answer. Well, I am going to let it go because I know my readers, such as you, will feel this answer may be more useful.

How do we measure the term of "Success"?

These days we measure success based on how much money we make, how big a house we have, what kind of car we have, what our job title is, and how many vacations we can take each year. These measures are superficial and so old fashioned and boring. For instance, I have seen some very wealthy patients who had the worst health and the worst relationships; I have seen someone who bought a costly car only to then pass away in 2 years; I have seen people who have a lot of money but did not have much common sense; I have seen people who worked very hard and saved a lot of money in the bank but who had no joy, no fun in their life; and, I have seen people who were not poor, had a good job but always worry about money. But some people do get it: they have money, and they have joy in their life, and these people I think have "true success."

What I think is "Success" (is measured differently) it is about the person's overall value, their happiness index, the long term results or outcome from their work, their inner harmony, their relationship with their family and others, their interest in continuous learning, their contributions to society, their mental and physical health, and their emotional balance. Don't get me wrong; people who are wealthy, have good jobs, own property, can also be in harmony, happy, healthy, contributing, and have good relationships when they have the skills which I mention next.

When you have the intent to achieve real "Success," you will be successful with your wealth, your relationships, your happiness, your career, and your health, etc.

How to reach this goal?

Here are some steps I call "Golden Tips," which worked perfectly for me; that's why I want to share them with you.

Know yourself, be yourself, do yourself, learn yourself.

You know yourself better than anyone (I assume. If not, you'd better ask your parents). You know your strengths, your weaknesses, what you like or don't like, your passion, your skill, your personality, and your dreams. You have your unique character, individual strength, and special ability. Just be yourself, people may like your uniqueness. If they don't like you, it is their problem, not your problem. If you try to be like other people, you lose your uniqueness, but you can always learn some good things from other people.

When you know your passion and strength, or the things you are best at doing, you will know how to find the right work in which you will be willing to learn, ready to devote yourself, and then you will be better and better from the sum of your experiences. Sometimes people may pursue something that is not truly their passion; they may try, become confused, and not know what to do. It is like being at a crossroads and not knowing which way to go. At this point, listen to your inner voice, your inner voice will guide you to make the right choices. Even if you chose a path that is not your passion, you might still be ok, because you may like it after trying it and learning it. You may have found a different passion. Listen to your inner voice, follow your gut, go with your heart, then put effort into your work, you may then blossom like a brilliant flower. You can achieve anything in your dreams, and you can bring abundance not only financially, but also in happiness. But to get there requires tremendous work, effort, learning, re-learning, and often learning from mistakes.

But you need to be aware of what is realistic or not realistic. Idealist may not be practical. For example, you want to start a business, but your financial situation is not right for starting a business. What should you do? You will need to take a more comprehensive view. Have a Plan A, and Plan B. Plan A is you succeed with your limited budget; Plan B is you fail with the original plan, but you have an alternative idea. This way, you are prepared for both outcomes. Some people try to get loan to start a business which in some cases is useful if you have a well-thought-out plan and have a Plan B. For others who don't have a well-thought-out plan or even a plan B when you fail, you will be burdened carrying a big loan which is like carrying a big heavy load on your shoulder until you cannot breathe anymore. When that happens, you may become sick, even develop a severe disease. My suggestion is that you need to prepare for both positive or negative outcomes mentally. Prepare financial funding for the business to cover at least the first year's expenses. And have a well thought out business plan that includes ideas about how to compete. Lastly, very important, you need to know how to save and be frugal. If you have profits, put them back into the business. Don't spend like a millionaire because you are not a millionaire. You are a beginner.

Success begins with an idea that could be your own or is inspired by others. When the idea becomes stronger, you start to research to find out if your plan is achievable or not. You then begin to put it into action, and from your activity, you accumulate experience. This experience includes learning, observing, trying, revising, modifying, and maturing. It is from within you this purpose came, and it is you who will make this plan a reality.

Any job or work involves learning, and it doesn't matter which job is the best. As long as you enjoy the work, this job is good (for you). If the job you love doesn't bring in enough money to pay the bills, you can always find a second job to supplement your income. This way, you can still have the work you love. If you complain that your job doesn't bring in enough or say people don't pay you enough even though you like what you do, you are displaying your negative energy, and this negative energy does not add anything; it only takes away from your joy.

If you are not sure about what you like or what you don't like to do, you may need to try different kinds of jobs to experience them; then, you may be able to decide about your ideal position or work. There is nothing wrong with trying different types of work. You will learn a lot, and you may discover some truth about yourself.

Most people think a high-paying job is a good job, and a low-paying job is a lousy job. But if you are dissatisfied with the "money job," you may become sick after a while. If you enjoy the work, you may be able to do it for a lifetime. Therefore, you would never be short of money. I met several patients and students who had changed their "Ideal job," "big money-making job," to a job they enjoyed doing. The bottom line is you need to do what is right for you.

No matter what other people passionately tell you, you can use their suggestions as a reference; but ultimately, the decision is up to you.

Sometimes you do a job that is not the work you like doing, but you have to pay the bills, feed the family, and make a living. In this case, you need to understand the law of nature, "The Yin, and the Yang," which means everything has two sides: good or bad. You may try to find the good parts of your work and focus on only the good parts. This way, you change your energy.

I always teach my students: You do nothing, you learn nothing, then you get nothing; you do something you learn something, and then you get something.

Here is one Daoist story:

A little mouse asked the sky, "You are so big and all the way up there and fear nothing; I am so little and fear everything. Can you give me some courage to live without fear?" The sky replied, "I have fear too, I am afraid of clouds. The clouds can block my Sun." The little mouse then asked the clouds, "Dear cloud, you are amazing and fear nothing, you can block the Sun. You must be the best." The cloud said, "I am not the best; I am afraid of the wind. When the wind comes, it blows me away." The little mouse then goes and asks the wind, "Dear wind, you are the best and strongest. You can blow the clouds away. Can you give me some courage?" The wind said, "No, I can blow the clouds away, but I am afraid of the wall because the wall can block me. Therefore, the wall is stronger than me." The little mouse went to see the wall and asks, "dear wall, you are the greatest one who can block the wind. You are perfect". The wall said, "No, I am not perfect. I am afraid of the little mouse. The little mouse can make a hole in my body, and then I can be broken from the holes." Finally, the little mouse understands and realized his self-value: be happy, be content, be satisfied, be himself.

Ability to deal with difficulties, willingness to face challenges.

If everything goes smoothly, there are no difficulties; you may not be learning many essential life skills. Through many challenges and overcoming obstacles, you learn and explore, keep learning, you try to figure things out, you then improve by making adjustments or changes. This is how you become smarter and smarter each year.

I've seen many people quit a dream, goal, or project they wanted to do when they encountered difficulties. They say, "this is not working." It may or may not be accurate. If you have tried, researched, consulted professionals, and done the best you can, but still failed, it may not be the right thing for you. But if you quit before making these efforts, you lose any chance of winning.

When you're just starting out, there is a lot to learn about doing business. Your passion or dream is an idea, but to make the concept become a reality, you need to know how to make it happen. Again, it involves researching and learning from all different perspectives much more than any specialized professional skill. I had no idea how to do business in the first year I had my clinic, but I took many courses, consulted professionals, read many books, and tried to talk to business people.

Most importantly, practice being honest, modest, patient, and observant, then people may be willing to help you and teach you. You may also create some good business connections at the same time.

Keep in mind that no matter what you do, there will always be difficulties. Having the ability to deal with challenges is not a genetic gift. It is a learned skill that can help you in many ways in life, work, and leisure. Most people prefer not to have challenges, but whoever is willing to take on challenges learns much more, gains much more.

How and where can we learn? Here are some tips for you:

First, you need determination. If you know this is the right thing to do after your education, work, and life experience, you need to drive forward with purpose. Just like Steve Jobs, his resolution made him the most famous person in the Computer world. (I don't mean you have to be famous). I made up a name for this kind of determination; I call it "Positive type OCD." OCD is an abbreviation for obsessive-compulsive disorder. Regular OCD is different; it is a condition diagnosed by a doctor, and it is not particularly valuable. But "Positive type OCD" is useful and productive and can help you succeed, to reach your dream, to achieve your goals.

Second, you need to be willing to learn and keep a positive mindset. Nothing comes easily, but things do become more manageable along the way while trying, experimenting, doing, and researching. You should not become negative over each little setback. Learning from challenges, trying to figure things out, you become smarter every day.

Third, be patient, there is no quick fix. Everything takes time, including solving problems. Don't expect that the next day everything will be ok (maybe it will, perhaps it won't). Use the time to do research, to figure it out, to find ways to overcome challenges. When you have patience, wisdom arises.

Nurture your growth mindset, continuous learning, and your efforts.

There are two kinds of people: those with a growth mindset, and those with a fixed mindset.

The person with a growth mindset does not limit himself, does not judge, does not go with the majority, or do as others say. His mind is open, his creativity is alive, his learning never stops, and he sees criticism positively and can ignore it if the criticism is too negative, or the person who is making the negative comments does not have good intentions. He doesn't judge; he keeps learning no matter how many people praise him. He does not stop even though he has achieved a certain level. He continues to grow, to improve, and to advance himself.

The fixed mindset is the majority, and it is normal. The person who has a fixed mindset always follows the trend, buys what other people buy, does what other people do, and goes with the majority. He is happy with praise but is unhappy or feels distressed with criticism; he may defend himself from the criticism trying to prove he is right, and he is smart. He judges people, judges other's work, projects, events, etc. He is not likely to grow and improve much beyond a certain point.

We all sometimes hear praise or applause when we achieve or do something good. Most people love to hear praise, which makes them feel good, happy, and feeling like they have value. The person who has a growth mindset doesn't need to revel in this kind of superficial admiration. Instead, he uses it as a stepping stone for further improvement, which helps him to achieve the next goal or to get to the next level.

Either mindset is fine; it just shows how different kinds of character create different results. Some people have good grades in school, but don't do that well in their work; some people have average grades in school but do very well, and it shows in their work. The kind of mindset you have plays a significant role in your performance.

But, if you are happy with what you do, that is all that matters. It's not necessary to be called "Successful." Your happiness is a big part of being successful.

I always believed that learning should be part of life, no matter how old or how young you are. Knowledge is an "intellectual investment." Open-minded and continuous learning can help your life in so many ways: health, career, personal relationships, emotional health, etc.

In my teaching, I always tell my students, "Keep learning; the day when you stop learning is the day you are doomed." I told my family the same thing, no matter if they listen or not.

What I call continuous learning is more than just going to school year after year, to get good grades and to get awards. Learning comes in many forms such as: going to school and learning form teachers, reading (most important) various books, attending conferences or lectures, group discussions, observing, listening, talking to people about things you are interested in, trying, going to random classes, researching stuff on the internet, doing things, watching educational shows or movies, and experimenting. While learning, keep your mind open, and have a non-judgmental attitude, you will learn faster. You may not notice it during your learning, but down the road, you will realize the path you are on is becoming easier and more comfortable, you will view things with a broader perspectives, you will then become more appreciative of your efforts on your learning journey.

Learning does not have any age limit. For younger people, you are creating opportunities for your future success; for older people, learning helps to prevent brain aging. Learning also helps you maintain your emotional stability. Everyone can learn and can improve, and everyone has the potential to grow as long they are open to learning.

The more you learn, the more comprehensive the understanding you will have. Knowledge is valuable, and experience is the voyage. When I was young, I always liked to be around people who had varied knowledge. I loved to listen to their stories, news, and their way of doing things. Making changes is also part of learning. You experience a change and find a new way of looking at things; with this, you can make improvements. People are taught in a certain way and continue this way generation after generation, and they lose their chance to try something different, something better.

Your effort is the motor of your success. If you have any ability, put 102% into your effort. That 2% extra may surprise you and may lead you to success. You won't lose anything if you do extra; the extra may bring you results, reputation, knowledge, and wisdom.

Many people don't take criticism well. There are different kinds of criticism: blaming or pointing out mistakes. Blaming is negative; pointing out mistakes, or errors, or giving suggestions is positive. Either way helps us to be better: getting blamed for something, makes us consider how we might stop the blaming; hearing about our mistakes can help us to see things from a wider angle and help us to improve. Therefore, criticism is a not bad thing; it is a warning light, a reminder, that allows us to re-adjust ourselves by making some changes or corrections. We don't see ourselves very well; other people can see us more than we see ourselves. Respect criticism, respect the person who is willing to point your weaknesses because only a true friend is willing to sacrifice the relationship to tell us the truth that we may not want to hear. It took me years to realize this wisdom, and now I appreciate it when others are willing to tell me the truth.

Knowing our weaknesses is where we can start to make corrections, then our effort to make improvements leads us to the next level. If we don't know our faults or are not willing to listen to others calling attention to them, there is no way we can work on them.

Your observation skill.

Observation is a skill; it is part of our growing and learning skills. Whatever we do and whatever we participate in, we need to pay attention to it. Observe how others talk, listen to what they say, observe their body language, and the level of their emotion, this is a part of learning. During a conversation, you may find some people have the knowledge that we need. They may have a different kind of energy; they may have gone through a lot in the past so that they may have an emotional imbalance. Or, they may be our inspiration.

Have you ever met people who cannot seem to stop talking? Nothing can get into their heads; they don't listen, don't learn, or don't know how to pay attention and observe. But if they put their mind into this kind practice, they may find out how beneficial it is to their life, work, and making friends.

"Respond; don't react. Listen; don't talk. Think; don't assume."
--------- *Raji Lukkoor*

"If you are mentally somewhere else, you miss real life."
-------- *Byron Katie*

Your confidence, patience, persistence, and self-control.

Being confident is not the same as being conceited. One is positive and attracts people, and one is negative and pushes people away.

Confidence comes from constant learning, observing, and practicing.

Confidence is not the same as "arrogance." Confidence is positive; arrogance is negative. I was arrogant in the past, but once I realized this was a weakness, I made an effort to change gradually, and I have changed. Studying Daoist philosophy has helped me very much on this journey.

Don't be afraid of criticism; don't let criticism take away your confidence. You can ignore it if the criticism does not make sense, or use it as a warning sign or reminder to yourself; there is no need to argue. Say less, do more, you will always get results.

Be patient, nothing in your character will change in a day, or an hour, good things take time. If you have a bad day or a bad year, it does not mean the next day or the next year will be the same. Everything will change, and your luck will change too.

Be persistent; don't give up so quickly. When things don't work now, it does not mean it won't work in the next year or next five years. As long as you continue to learn and do the best you can, you will succeed at some point. Use your intuition and wisdom to figure out why things are not working, make changes if necessary.

Self-control is another way to say discipline. This is something many average people are lacking. Ordinary people may not have the goals you have. Therefore, the mindful practice of self-control can make you stand out and succeed. Self-control is crucial as it relates to food, drink, activities, lifestyle, talking, doing things, emotions, etc. By avoiding extremes, things are less likely to go awry. Many people fail, and part of the reason is they lack self-control.

Your demeanor, kindness, and generosity.

This part may not look like it has much to do with "Success." But in fact, and it is an integral part of achieving success.

Everything we do has consequences: good or bad. We will see good consequences if we do good things, and we will see terrible consequences if we do bad things. Unfortunately, many people don't think about the "consequences" before they start doing something. For instance, if you were upset and had a loud fight with your co-worker (you did not know the right way to communicate at that time), the next thing you know, you might get laid off. For drug users, they look for temporary pleasure, but the consequences are massive, including possible death. In diet, we eat what we enjoy but don't consider that certain foods can cause illness. Later, when heart disease or diabetes occurs, we realize, oops, too bad.

If we pay attention to demeanor, kindness, and generosity, we will not hurt another person's feelings; we will not take advantage of other people. We would provide help when others need it, and we would respect others and their work, and we will have less stress in our own life using these positive practices.

Your character, kindness, demeanor, and following ethical codes attracts others and makes it easier for you to make friends. In our modern world, friendship, relationship, and connections are essential. When you need information, a job, a research grant, or anything you may need help with, some of your friends may be able to help you or guide you.

Any "Success" must include a moral code. If money comes from fraud, cheating, taking advantages of others, or destroying nature, I don't call this real success. I can only say the money is from greediness or dirty money. A moral code needs to be part of our work ethic and practiced daily.

Keep your word; don't promise something if you cannot deliver. If you put yourself in the same situation: someone promised you but cannot do it, what would you think and feel?

In personal relationships, if the relationship isn't working, there must be a reason. There is no need to be upset or force the relationship. You will find the right partner if your mind is in the right place. If you have a lover or someone close to you, you should not hurt her or him using your nasty words. Don't think, "it is ok to be rude; she/he understands me." This is very selfish and can destroy a relationship. You want to plant "love seeds," not "hate seeds."

Be modest; listen to others. Don't try to show off. No matter how good you think are, there is always someone better than you. Be open to learning, be humble; you will be better every year. Learn to praise other people; you send good energy to other people who will feel great hearing your positive comments.

When working with others, you may not like certain things or specific ways of doing things, but you may have to accept it because not everything is about you, your wants, your needs. We all have "likes and dislikes," but we practice acceptance because there are many ways to do things, and we may learn from doing something a "different way," I call it looking for the bright side of everything. There are many colors in our life. A color you don't like could be a color someone else likes.

Remove "revenge" from your living dictionary. Revenge is very harmful; it can only make you sicker and unhappy. Forgiveness is the way to get you out of any dark emotion.

Whatever you do, make sure to check the regulations, laws, and whatever legal requirement. If not, you may jeopardize your work and waste your time, and eventually, you have to deal with so much trouble, unpleasant tasks, which all lead to unhappiness and depression. I have seen some people going through these experiences, and it's not fun.

The Mind and thought process.

Our mind plays a vital role in our life, wellbeing, and success. The mind is the highest power and relates to everything we do, and we work for. Our mind and thought process can guide us along the path to achievement, but also can take us to a wrong path, leading to failure. If our mind is weak, we can be easily be dragged into what I call "the box," "doing/acting/thinking that is controlled by others." If our mind is strong and healthy, we have internal strength. We are rooted, balanced; we cannot be influenced by outside forces, unhealthy recommendations, or trends that everyone may be following.

We should not blame others for their mistakes, but instead, check ourselves to see what we can do to make things better. We need to find ways to solve problems we encounter at work and in life and avoid the same mistakes in the future. We should be willing to work on ourselves and be ready to make changes, willing to accept criticism and let it be our reminder for future improvement. We need to see things from a wider angle and listen to other's opinions, including those that may be the opposite of ours. We should try to respect one another no matter what social or financial level, and try not to criticize others. We should try to praise others for their good work, kind personality, or whatever good quality a person may have. We feel good doing so, and we need to continue to have this kind of practice throughout our lifetime.

Having a strong mind is not the same as being stubborn and rigid; the strong mind I describe here means balanced, healthy, organized, open to differences, and logical. A stubborn or inflexible mind is far from balanced and can prevent you from advancement.

Don't haggle over trifles, which I call being "small-minded," focusing on small things. But you do need to pay attention to important things which are meaningful in your life and career. Losing a few dollars does not hurt you; losing your health/career/life can hurt you. There is a Chinese proverb we used to hear, "Don't pick up a sesame seed but throw away a watermelon," obviously a sesame seed is a lot smaller than a watermelon.

Different people think differently, and different kinds of thinking produce different energy. It is not about right or wrong, just differences. Here is a Daoist story:

Three men are walking on the street after a rainstorm. They pass a wall that is wet on the bottom half of the wall. A little ant is crawling up the wall, but the ant keeps falling because the wall is wet. The little ant keeps trying climb up, falls down, again climbs up, then again falls down. The first man looked at this ant and made this comment he said: "This is a stupid little ant, he knows that he cannot get up there but still climbs, how dumb he is." The second man also made a comment he said: "Yes, I agree with you, he is stupid; if it was me, I'd go around to find a dry place then it would be so much easier to climb up to the top of the wall." The third person thought a moment, then said: "This ant is not stupid, he is brave, persistent, he does not give up even though he fails many times. He will get there eventually. We humans should do better than an ant, right? I am inspired by this little ant".

The story is simple, but it relates to our being surrounded by different people with different energy.

For many years, people work primarily to make a living, raise children, pay bills. Nothing wrong with this. But if you want to achieve, to reach your goal, you will need to do things differently. In the beginning, don't just calculate how much money you can make, how many benefits you can get. You should think, "How much can I learn from this job? What are my long-term goals"? With this mindset, you will achieve.

If you would like to know more about the relationship between the mind and diseases, please refer to the book written by Dr. Catherine Kurosu and myself. "True Wellness, The Mind," published in July 2019.

Your Understanding of "Balance."

In every book I wrote, there are always numerous references to the word "Balance." After years of practicing preventive medicine, I know that balance is a big part of human health and success.

I have seen people who are "very successful," who made a lot of money, owned a lot of property, but have poor health; some divorced several times; some were in the hospital saying, "life is not fair, I worked so hard, but now I cannot enjoy my life." Some of them passed away relatively young. What they didn't understand was the fundamental principle: "Balance in everything": balanced work, emotion, exercise, eating, social, talking or conversation, traveling, etc.

Daoist philosophy emphasizes balance, simplicity, be who you are, harmony, and going with the flow. This does not mean you can sit in the house doing nothing, have no concerns, and everything will be provided. It is regarding the flow of your ambition, your passion, what you are drawn to, what you'd like to create, produce, your talent, and making something happen as a result of your work. If you don't understand Daoist philosophy, you would not know how to go with the flow.

Your work needs to be balanced, not too much, not too little. Younger people can work more hours than older people, but they need to know at what point they need to stop working and rest. I once argued with my cousin, who used to be a translator at the United Nations, as he made some comments about struggling with his work after he reached the age of 60. He said his brain was not as sharp as before; his translation was slower than before. I did not believe him at that time; I was convinced that if we try hard to do things for our health, we will not lose any of our faculties. But sure enough, when I reached age 62, I realized it is a reality that we all have to accept. Trying to do the right things such as eating well, exercising regularly, getting enough rest, and keeping your mind active helps but cannot necessarily keep you as sharp as you were in your youth. I realized I needed to cut back on my work, take better care of my body, and balance my life.

A balanced life involves doing everything in moderation: drinking, eating, partying, socializing, housework, conversations, activities, travel, and exercise. It is not about trying to have a perfect life; it is about maintaining a happy and healthy life.

Being organized.

I have always struggled with my organizational skills, by continually working to improve this skill, I have made much improvement, and this has brought me much convenience. I had my business since 1996, and I found the organizational capability to be essential.

First of all, we need to learn how to keep track of things, not to rely on others keeping track for us because others may not be able to do it well or may forget to do it. When this happens, we are stuck. This can also help us to avoid being taken advantage of by others, such as over-paying bills, like an error caused by the telephone company. I have seen insurance companies take advantage of people who are weak or not able to keep track. My own experience had taught me a lesson too. In this fast-paced society, not many people are willing to spend the extra time to look over things thoroughly, and this certainly allows scammers to take advantage. It takes time to keep track of things, but it is definitely worth the effort.

Keeping track of time is another thing we need to watch. If you are late once nobody would take it too seriously, but if you are late or forget what time you are supposed to meet someone, this can hurt your reputation. I have noticed that some people don't read emails carefully even though they are well educated; they did not pay attention to the date on an email. My suggestion is to write down which day, what date, and what time, you don't want to have to rely on your memory about appointments because it's easy to forget.

If you are good with computers, using technology to help you keep track of things is very helpful. But not everyone is good with a computer, and there are other ways to help keep track of things: such as a reliable filing system, know where to put your stuff, use labeling, in an organized way. If you practice "simplicity," you then have less to worry about, and it's easier to keep track of things.

Next, get in the habit of writing things down. Keep a note pad with you all the time. Write down the work you have to do in order: urgent, most important, important, semi-important, next day work, less important but needs to be done at some point, weekly work, monthly work, yearly work, etc.

If you want to become an author in the future, start writing a journal or diary. I regret that I did not keep a journal, I thought I could remember, but I did not. This cost me a lot of time in trying to get back these memories and experiences from my brain, friends, classmate, family, and others. The memory storage in our mind can only hold a certain amount of memories, and over a period of time, some memories leak out. But if you have a journal or diary, it can help bring back a memory. Even a short sentence can help to bring a memory back.

Periodically clean your drawers, files, overloaded paperwork, you may find something you were looking for, and this also helps you to remove some junk or things you no longer need.

Keeping your word or promises is part of training for your sincerity. If you cannot deliver, you should not make a promise. It is tough to work with someone who cannot keep their word or promise. Also, their chance of being promoted is much less. If you cannot do something you promised, you should tell the truth about it. People will appreciate at least hearing the truth.

If you have a job requiring that you work certain hours each day, you should be on time. Even better, you should arrive to work 5 to 15 minutes earlier and leave work 5 to 15 minutes later. Being there earlier helps you to get organized for the day, both mentally and physically. Even though you have the right to leave at the exact time, it is better to leave work after the precise time. This shows you want to get your work done, you care, and you don't mind contributing a bit extra of your time. This extra time can help you to organize your time, finish your work, clear your mind, calm down, and relax a little before you head out on the road back home. If you had some stress one day and then rush home, your risk of having an accident could be higher than average.

When something happens where you are either late for work or have to leave early, you can explain your situation, which everyone understands for rare cases. If you want to keep your job, it is better not to have this kind of excuse often.

Your strategic work.

A person with a chaotic or dysfunctional mind, or ADD (attention deficit disorder), would have difficulty succeeding, but it is not impossible. For example, you may want to do many things because you have many interests, or you start working on many projects at once. Later you realize you are overwhelmed and not able to accomplish your work. The good news is that you can work efficiently and achieve your goals through training, learning, discipline, and practice. It is all about focus.

First of all, work on intelligent communication in which the conversation is logical, to the point, sequential (not back froth or circular), and non-repeating. Communication needs to be very clear and include respect. Try to avoid conversations that carry emotion, which often goes nowhere, sometimes making the conversation go in a negative circle. If you have questions or are making a statement, keep your items short and precise, get to the point. Try not to assume other people will know what you mean (which I did in the past, but I am better now), because people cannot read your mind (nobody can). During open discussions, don't be afraid to ask questions; it doesn't matter if it's a "good question" or "bad question." People who have a judgmental mind make this assumption about "good questions, or bad questions." Any question is a good question, no matter what. When someone gives the answer you needed, don't forget to say "thank you, that helps." We often forget to say thank you, even though we do appreciate it. But that "Thank you" makes other people feel good, and we want to make people feel good, not make people feel bad. When everyone feels good, the work can get done quicker and better. Kindness connects people.

I hear this a lot, "I will do it tomorrow," "I will do it next week." Then tomorrow comes, and they may say the same thing because they forgot. Don't wait for tomorrow if you can do it today. There will always be some other work that needs to be done the next day, the following week. Doing it today, or now, definitely helps to get the job done. In the past, I said the same thing "I will do it tomorrow or next week." After several months the work was still there. This is why I changed my strategy: "get it done and get over it." Now I always get whatever work needs to be done "done."

If you want something or want to achieve something, you will need to first map this out in your mind. You can "look at" this map and think about how you can do what is necessary to get what you want. If you have the negative thought, "I will never get what I want," you have already told yourself to give up. If you have positive thoughts, work toward the place on your "map," and keep going until you get there.

Here is my experience from when I lived in Massachusetts. The first time when I was visiting Boston (maybe 1989 or 1990), we went to the Public Garden and the Boston Common, I loved Boston, and I especially fell in love with those condos next to the Boston Common on Tremont St. I told myself in a kind of wishful thinking, "someday I am going to live there, just to experience the one of the best locations in Boston downtown." My husband told me that those are some of the most expensive condos in Boston because of the location; we definitely cannot afford to own that property. Somehow that wish was always stuck in my mind............ I finally did get a condo in a building next to the Common in 2008, a very small condo, but my wish was granted, and we enjoyed it for nine years.

I always wanted to live in the South because I don't like cold weather, and the cold weather affects my health. I kept telling myself, "Someday I will move South." I kept thinking this way for about ten years. I am now living in Florida, a beautiful place with perfect weather that has helped my health.

I won, I got what I wanted. But this is not all from luck, and I had to give up the business I spent all my energy on building in Massachusetts. It was not easy, but I got my balance. From the Daoist philosophy that everything has two sides, the Yin and the Yang, I got my balance: I lose some, and I gain some more.

Some people see failure as a terrible thing, and they can lose their health and fall into depression. Failure is just a part of learning on our journey, it is reasonable, and there is no such thing as "never failing" anyway. Going through failure, you gain a lot of wisdom and insight, your work improves, you're smarter, can avoid mistakes, and you move closer to achievement.

When you meet new people for whatever reason, you want to connect with people. Trying to have a pleasant conversation but try not to talk about your business or your talent; try to listen to other people. Later, when people get to know you and like you, they may ask you for your name card or ask what you do. This is when you can tell people what you do, what you sell, but don't try to make any suggestion or to ask people to buy your product or come for your service. Always strive to build the connection first. No matter how hard you try to sell, try to convince others, it won't work if people don't know you. Connect with them with small stories, be a good listener, let others talk. Be humble. When people ask you what you do, this is the perfect time to give your name card. Once people know you and like you, your chance to do business with them is better.

Time is valuable and precious. You can buy anything with your money, but you cannot buy time. If you waste your time, you lose your precious time. All of a sudden, you will realize you are older, you may wish you could have done something differently, or you may wish you had not done things you did in the past. When you get to the age where you realize that you are unable to do something like you did before, you feel terrible. It is better to cherish the precious time now; use it to learn, to create, to read, to have healthy social activities, to make connections, to exercise, to take care of yourself, to be with your family, to enjoy being with your friends, to work on and reach your dream, and to do things you enjoy doing. Don't waste time, because you can never get time back.

Teamwork is another essential quality in the workforce and a self-employed business. Any work involves working with people, but not everyone has good people skills. Working on your communication skills, your humility, your listening skill, your structured mind, your supportive attitude, and your kindness, you will earn people's trust and foster teamwork.

One more thing that is also important: Don't make any decision when you are emotional because you would often be making a wrong decision during a sensitive time. Once your emotion is stable, you will be able to look at the whole situation and be able to make a better choice or critical decision.

No matter what you do, how busy you are, don't forget to work on improving yourself. Many people have a habit of pointing fingers and often blame others for not doing a good job. But the brilliant ones never stop working on self-improvement, they don't blame, only learn. These smart ones will reach the highest point of life, which is the total happiness and optimum health. That is the Dao, that is the truth, and that is what I call the good life.

Chapter 21: Good Health, East Meets West

Since I have struggled with my health for most of my life, I cherish the time when my health problems are under control. I feel that my health is my wealth. I don't envy people who have just wealth or have a luxury lifestyle, but I do envy people who have good health. What I call good health is not only big muscles, a beautiful body, being strong physically. What I call good health is a healthy body, a bright and healthy mind, and a good spirit, a healthy attitude, good stamina, and all parts of the body being in balance and harmony. That's what I call real wealth. It is like gold, pure like spring water, strong like bamboo, and rooted like a mountain. This is true wellness. Am I close to it? I think so, but it's still a work in progress.

How can a person maintain good health? The commercial world has provided so many products, gadgets, apparatus, supplements, health classes, and health foods. Theoretically, we should all be in good health. But, no. Our health does not parallel these commercial offerings. Even with an abundance of suggested solutions, diseases of all kinds continue to appear.

One of my patients from out of state has been using many different kinds of medication but is still not feeling well. I asked him if he had checked the side effects of these medications. He said no, he said that his doctor monitors his blood for him. Many people are not aware that using drugs for a long time can cause unpleasant side effects even though their blood chemistry may seem normal. They assume it is safe if a doctor prescribes the medications. Yes and no, it depends on what kind of doctor: responsible or not responsible.

Medicine is great but not perfect. My friend Julie had anemia. Without knowing what caused her anemia, her doctor prescribed iron pills. To me, this is shooting an arrow blindfolded: you may hit the target, or may not hit it. It could do more harm than good in some instances. A good doctor would find out what caused the anemia, then address the cause or remove the cause so that the patient can heal naturally.

Everything has consequences, so do diseases and causes. If you are health conscious and mindful, and you do healthy things, you will have healthful consequences; if you have a mind not focused on health, and you do something that harms your health, you will have disease or experience unpleasant symptoms as a consequence. Generally speaking, the causes of illness have these factors: your mind, your attitude, your lifestyle (which includes eating habits and exercising correctly), and your prevention strategies. Very simple, but not so simple to some people.

In my own experience, in addition to working on self-improvement in mind and spirit, moving the body and exercising is crucial. The modern world is not healthy. We are continually aiming to make more profits, more investments, more of everything. It gets to the point people don't know how to breathe anymore. You wonder why so many people are cranky, use alcohol to deal with life, use drugs to de-stress, or go doctors to get more pills. We often forget that we have power. We, as individuals, must make an effort to change, to make the world a healthy world. If we understand the balance in life, work, and health, we will find a way to do it. I hear from my patients all the time, "I don't have any time to do exercise," but that is not true. Just 30 minutes of exercise a day can change your health. You can do activities that you like; there's no need to run 5 miles a day. Your intuition and awareness can guide you to choose the right exercise for your daily practice. I have been amazed to see many of my patients feel better just doing the exercises that I prescribed to them targeted to their illnesses, by regulating their diet, and managing their stress. They were able to use less medication even stopped completely; they feel better overall, and most important: they are happier.

Many of us go to doctors when we are sick, but very few pay attention to "prevention." Some people become so frustrated after suffering from some severe illness, but then realize they need to make some changes. On a 2019 trip to China, I was informed of the loss of a classmate, and also that some other friends almost died from severe illness.

When it comes to diseases, many of them are produced by ourselves. If we ask ourselves: am I happy or not happy? How is my diet? Is it balanced? How many cups of water do I drink? How is my sleeping? Do I do exercise daily? How is my emotional state in general? Do I get upset often? How do I deal with my stress? Do I deal with my stress healthily and logically? Am I an organized person? How is my relationship with my partner? How is my workload? How is my pain? Do I make time for myself?

After you write down the answers to these questions, you may realize that many of these things are connected or associated, and you may be able to make changes. With these changes, your life changes too. You have a choice to join the "rat race world" or enter the "balanced life world." It is not about which is better; it is a personal choice. The only difference is the consequences that you will be dealing with later in life.

We often ignore the relationship between stress and health. Among all illnesses, many are induced by stress. Chronic stress is the number one cause of diseases such as hypertension, heart disease, cholesterol problems, insomnia, digestive problems, weight problems, depression, anxiety, kidney disease, cancer, and more. We live in a modern world, and the contemporary world does create stress. The only way to avoid illness is to know how to manage stress.

First of all, we need to recognize what causes stress. Stress is everywhere, and we cannot avoid it. But we can find ways not to let stress harm us. When we feel stressed, it is because our body and our mind are responding to a situation in an anxious way. We may feel tense, tired, short of breath, headache, insomnia, our voice may become high pitched and loud, our tone sharp, aggressive, our face may turn red, our heartbeat is faster, BP is more elevated, we feel upset. This is the acute stage of stress I call the explosive type. You only hurt yourself with this dangerous type of stress; you may damage your relationships with others too. The worst part is: it does not help anything.

When stress is allowed to accumulate, then it becomes chronic stress that is harmful to our body and mind. When your body is tense for long periods, it affects blood flow and energy flow, and both are crucial to our health. If we can find a way to improve our response to external stresses, our body can be more naturally relaxed. Since we cannot change the situation, we can only change our response, finding a way to neutralize the situation as best we can, and then moving forward. This way, you can feel like you are just doing your work and not feel like you are being stressed. If the situation cannot be fixed right away, you may take a break or try to distance yourself from it temporarily. Later, you may find a new solution to the problem causing the stress. Stress may not always be a bad thing because we can learn something from the stress. And learning is positive.

Some tips that may help you to relieve your stress:

1. The right communication can be helpful. Language is an art; it is a living art, and we should all pay attention to it. Saying "I" versus "you" is a better way to communicate. We may use "I feel....", "I would like...", "I think...," "I may have....", "I could have....", "I hope..."... This way seems more modest. Pointing the finger at others is aggressive, critical, and less likely to solve problems. Speaking in a peaceful way enables the other party to respond to you peacefully. If you speak in a loud and aggressive voice, you are likely to trigger the other person to react the same way and cause fighting. There is enough fighting in this world; no need to create more fighting.

Not everyone is taught to know how to communicate the right way, but if you take a few deep breaths before you speak, your tone will be better. And with these deep breaths, you bring more oxygen to your brain; you may come up with some better words. Deep breathing is the first element of Qi Gong.

2.   We should also try to think of the other person or put ourselves in the other person's position, doing this, we can understand the person better. For instance, when you are trying to criticize someone, think about how you feel when someone is trying to criticize you, and what your reaction would be?

3.   Think of and appreciate the good things in your life during a stressful time, think of the people who love you, this may help you to get through difficult times. We all have had hard times at some point in our life, but think for a moment, we have more enjoyable things in our life than bad things. Compare this with people living in third world countries; we are in a much better situation than they are. Hard times can be compared to a storm that comes and goes. Therefore, there is no need to be obsessed with negatives when things don't go the way we want. Things will work out in the end.

4.   Drink a cup of tea to soothe your mind, especially Jasmine tea.

5.   Listen to some beautiful music, or listen to relaxation music. Music has a healing effect. You can also pick a song you like, sing, sing it loud. Singing is very good for you. It doesn't matter if you have a good voice or not. Singing loud opens your lung energy, exercises your voice, lifts your energy, and also lifts your spirit.

6.   Read a book, any book; this takes your mind away from stressful thoughts.

7.   Talk to your family or friends; don't be afraid to call them. If no one answers the phone, call another one, I am sure you will find someone to talk to. When you let things out, talk things through, feelings of stagnation are relieved.

8. Both Qi Gong and Tai Chi are great exercises for stress reduction, and immediate results can be felt. You can feel openness in your energy pathways and feel better right away.

If you don't want to do Qi Gong or Tai Chi, you can choose to walk, jog, play sports, go swimming, hike, ride a bike, travel, do yoga, lift weights, or other exercises.

9. You can do breathing exercises, breathe slowly, deeply, and with a focused mind. Meditation is a great way to relieve stress; even as little as five minutes can help.

10. Drink more water. Stress or other symptoms can be exacerbated when you are dehydrated. The brain contains water, more than 80%. When you are stressed, your brain may not be functioning at its best, which leads you to react to the stress poorly. Therefore, drinking more water helps to relieve stress.

Despite the rapid development of modern medicine, diseases have not decreased, and hospitals are busier than ever. It may be a good thing in terms of boosting the economy; medical institutions make a lot of money. But many patients are unable to pay large sums of money for treatment, or even lose their lives. It's unreasonable to complain about doctors when they can't cure you. Doctors are overworked, and some are unable to examine and accurately diagnose and treat each patient thoroughly. They can help with your symptoms, but they can't preserve your health. Western medicine is valuable in saving your life, relieving your symptoms, removing lumps, and treating wounds. Although diagnosis with western medicine has better examination tools, the accuracy of the diagnosis still depends on the quality of the individual doctors, their medical knowledge, and clinical experience. It's the same in China and the United States. Some small hospitals have excellent doctors, and it's not necessary to go to a big hospital, it all depends on the doctor's skill and kindness.

I have had many struggles with my health, including allergies. But no doctors advised me to get an allergy test to find out what I was allergic to. None advised me to see an allergy specialist. Finally, I decided to go to see an allergy specialist and get blood work done. That is how I found out I am allergic to many things. Not wanting to get allergy treatment because of the lengthy treatment time involved, at least now I can control my diet, which helps a lot. Relying on doctors to cure me seems hopeless. My health is in my own hands, my effort, my discipline, my knowledge, and my hard work.

I think Eastern medicine is more valuable in improving the quality of health and preventing disease. It is especially valuable in prevention. A major component of eastern medicine is maintaining harmony among the various parts of the body, the flow of energy, and the active coordination of the mind and body. If we know how to prevent, and aim to live our lives smarter and healthier, we can avoid unnecessary troubles. Here are my four suggestions:

1. First, exercise. No matter what kind of exercise you like, you need to do it every day. This way, you can keep your nervous system and your musculoskeletal system functioning normally. It also helps the organs to work properly. Challenge your lazy, undisciplined habits. It will become easier when you get into the habit of exercising. I like comprehensive exercises: tai chi, qigong, stretching, weight lifting, muscle strengthening, cycling, hiking, and so on. Tai chi, in particular, is excellent for mental and physical health.

2. Second, diet. Most of us know what is healthy and what is not. But many of us don't adjust our menus to what we know. This often leads to diabetes, high blood pressure, heart disease, fatty liver, obesity, high blood lipids, and even stroke.

3. Third, mindset. Positive thinking and a good attitude are essential factors for healing and prevention. We see and hear a lot of negativity, but we don't have to be dragged into it. We can't change others, but we can change ourselves, make our own lives more relaxed and happier.

4. Fourth, reduce stress. Modern life has given us a grand economic boost but also has reduced our precious time. Many of us are continually adding tension to our life. Learning to reduce stress makes life much more enjoyable. I've talked a lot about stress reduction previously. Learning to simplify our life is an excellent practice in stress management.

How to use Eastern and Western medicine most efficiently?

For any acute problems, we should choose western medicine unless you have a muscle sprain or other pain not involving a structural problem, in which case you can try acupuncture, herbal medicine, or Tui Na (massage) therapy.

For emotional problems, I do not recommend using medication because the medication's side effect may cause more harm to your body. Eastern medicine is the first choice, along with Qi Gong, Tai Chi, meditation, herbal medicine, diet change, nutrition support, etc.

For ongoing or chronic problems, you should choose eastern medicine, especially Qi Gong. A well-trained Qi Gong teacher has good Qi Gong knowledge, which can be very helpful. You can also try acupuncture, Tui Na therapy, herbal therapy, nutrition support, etc. I have seen many patients who were lacking proper nutrition due to their busy schedules.

Don't ignore the power of Qi Gong. Qi Gong is under-rated for its excellent healing benefits. I have so many stories where using Qi Gong helped a patient's healing. Because of the shortage of quality Qi Gong teachers, the popularity of Qi Gong is low. Because of this, I decided to do training for Qi Gong therapists soon. This way, more and more people may be helped most gently. We often say, "No pain, no gain." But in Qi Gong healing, it's "No pain yes gain." This certainly improves the quality of life.

To put it simply; life is short, and we must cherish and embrace every minute.

Final Words

Why do I write and work so hard? I do not want to compete with others, nor do I want to make a lot of money. I don't want to lead an extravagant life. What I wanted when I was young was unattainable, and when I came to America, no one controlled my ideas, no one stopped me from doing what I wanted to do. To be fulfilled, I must work hard to create a new vision, a mission, a new set of values, and a life full of happiness. Every stage in life has a different focus and set of choices. In my next phase, I'm going to focus on how to live a lighter, simpler life and keep trying to fulfill my mission, which is to let more people benefit from natural medicine and natural therapy. This helps to make people more appreciative of the value of life, their physical and mental health, friendship, and true love. It also discourages greed, ego, self-abuse, selfishness, and unlimited desire. Only by simplifying can we gain more time, energy, and protect our body and mind. Our brains will also be more alert, logical, and less likely to age prematurely.

Life is a path we all follow, and it is not always a smooth path. Life is like a mountain, with hills, rocks, obstacles, thorns, broken trees, and many unexpected obstacles. We can't let these obstacles interfere with our life. We have to keep moving forward, moving beyond or removing barriers, endeavoring to reach the peak or top of the mountain. We should be content and happy with what we have and who we are, and be comfortable with ourselves. We keep connections with our friends and family, no matter whether they live near or far.

We need to protect our physical and emotional health and allow our good health to accompany us on our life journey. When we reach the end of our life path, we can say to ourselves; I did what I thought was best, I enriched my life with experiences, I am satisfied with my experience, I have lived a happy life. I will leave this world happy, and my spirit will continue.

A good life does not come easily but comes from how we build and create it.

We create our life by knowing how to love each other as well as how to love ourselves and nourish our body, mind, and soul. We give, we cherish, and we embrace; we maintain internal peace, inner strength, and mindfully use our wisdom. We have many good friends, both old and new. We have plenty of good food and a cheerful spirit. We have our passions, our mission, and our cause. We are not afraid of facing challenges, and we know going through the challenges helps us to become stronger. We continue to explore and to experience life, to feel it, and to learn from it, to give, to embrace all we have, and who we are with. We aim to protect our Mother Earth, nature, and our land. Together, we can create a peaceful and beautiful world.

☐

My Family:

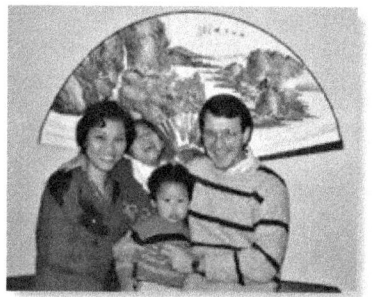
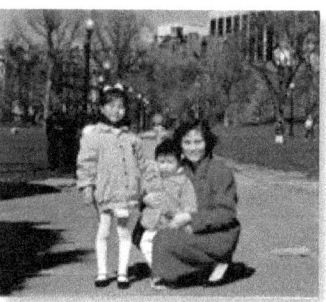

1. Milford, MA 1989
2. Boston, MA 1990

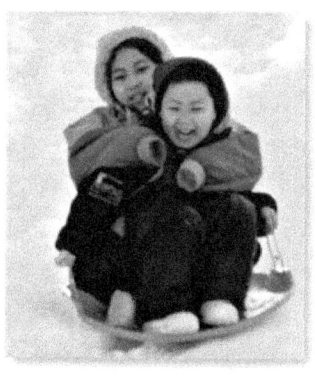
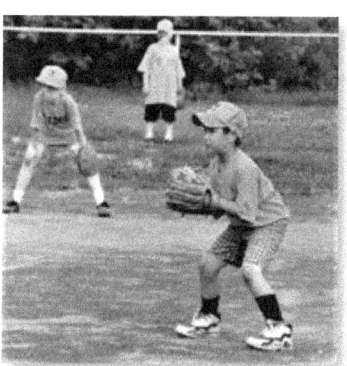

3. Milford, MA front yard hill
4. Milford, MA little league

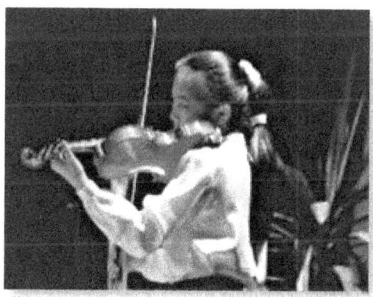
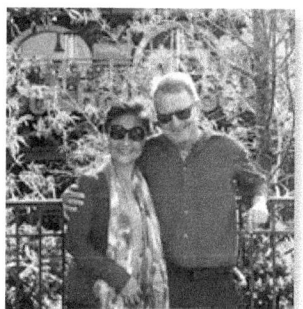

5. Sharon's solo
6. Florida 2019

Dr. Aihan Kuhn's Books

Natural Healing with Qi Gong
(Published in 2004)
Simple Chinese Medicine
(Published in 2009)
Award-winning Book
Tai Chi for Depression
(Published in 2017)
Nominated for Best Book Award
Tai Chi in 10 Weeks
(Published in 2017)
Nominated for Best Book Award
Brain Fitness
(Published in 2017)
Nominated for Best Book Award
True Wellness
(Published in 2018)
Award-winning Book, three awards
True Wellness, The Mind
(Published in 2019)
True Wellness, The Heart
To be released (2020)
Qi Gong for Travelers
(Published in 2013)
Weight Loss the Natural Way
(Published in 2014)

Dr. Aihan Kuhn's Home Study Programs:

1. Learning Tai Chi in 10 Weeks
2. Natural Healing with Qi Gong
3. Brain Fitness Program
4. Chinese Medicine for Self-Healing
5. Qi Gong for Cancer Healing
6. Tai Chi for Emotion Balance
7. Tai Chi for Seniors
8. And more

Website: www.draihankuhn.com

www.ingramcontent.com/pod-product-compliance
Lightning Source LLC
Chambersburg PA
CBHW071353210526
45465CB00001B/74